# THE AUTHOR

Rosemary Conley is the UK's leading diet and fitness expert and has sold over five million books and almost three million videos on the subject.

Together with her husband, Mike Rimmington, Rosemary runs three companies: Rosemary Conley Diet and Fitness Clubs, which operates a national network of almost 200 franchises running over 2,000 classes weekly; Quorn House Publishing Ltd, which publishes Rosemary Conley Diet & Fitness magazine with a circulation of around 250,000; and Rosemary Conley Enterprises.

Rosemary appears regularly on television and radio and has had her own TV series on BBC, ITV and satellite channels.

Rosemary has a daughter, Dawn by her first marriage, and Rosemary, Mike and Dawn are all committed Christians.

## ALSO BY ROSEMARY CONLEY

*Rosemary Conley's Hip and Thigh Diet*

*Rosemary Conley's Complete Hip and Thigh Diet*

*Rosemary Conley's Inch Loss Plan*

*Rosemary Conley's Hip and
Thigh Diet Cookbook* (with Patricia Bourne)

*Rosemary Conley's Metabolism Booster*

*Rosemary Conley's Whole Body Programme*

*Rosemary Conley's New Hip and
Thigh Diet Cookbook* (with Patricia Bourne)

*Shape Up for Summer*

*Rosemary Conley's Beach Body Plan*

*Rosemary Conley's Flat Stomach Plan*

*Be Slim! Be Fit!*

*Rosemary Conley's New Body Plan*

*Rosemary Conley's New Inch Loss Plan*

*Rosemary Conley's Low Fat Cookbook*

*Rosemary Conley's Red Wine Diet*

*Rosemary Conley's Low Fat Cookbook Two*

*Eat Yourself Slim*

*Rosemary Conley's Gi Jeans Diet*

*Rosemary Conley's Step By Step Low Fat Cookbook*

# Rosemary Conley's
# COMPLETE FLAT STOMACH PLAN

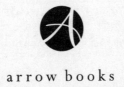

arrow books

Reissued by Arrow Books in 2002

5 7 9 10 8 6

Copyright © Rosemary Conley Enterprises 1996

First published in the United Kingdom in 1996 by Arrow Books

The Random House Group Limited
20 Vauxhall Bridge Road, London, SW1V 2SA

Random House, Australia (Pty) Limited
20 Alfred Street, Milsons Point, Sydney,
New South Wales 2061, Australia

Random House New Zealand Limited
18 Poland Road, Glenfield, Auckland 10, New Zealand

Random House (Pty) Limited
Isle of Houghton, Corner of Boundary Road & Carse O'Gowrie,
Houghton 2198, South Africa

The Random House Group Limited Reg. No. 954009

www.randomhouse.co.uk

A CIP catalogue record for this book is available
from the British Library

Papers used by Random House are natural, recyclable products made from wood grown in sustainable forests. The manufacturing processes conform to the environmental regulations of the country of origin

ISBN 978 0 09 944163 2 (from Jan 2007)
ISBN 0 09 944163 2

Printed and bound in Great Britain by
Bookmarque Ltd, Croydon, Surrey

# Contents

This nutritionally sound programme encapsulates all the latest scientific thinking on healthy eating and exercise and puts the message across in a positive, easy-to-follow and understandable way. It's not just a diet but a whole way of life that encourages you to make long-term changes to your lifestyle and reap optimum benefits for health.

*Dr Andrew Prentice,*
*Head of Energy Metabolism Research,*
*Dunn Clinical Nutrition Centre, Cambridge*

Anyone who is overweight and who follows the advice in this book will reduce their body weight and size. To maintain these benefits, the principles described need to be followed in the long term. Failure to do so may result in your regaining your lost weight.

From your interest in this book it is clear that you either have an interest in health, ot it is possible that you have an underlying problem with your eating habits. In extreme cases, this could manifest itself as an eating disorder which requires more help than this book can offer. In this instance, I would encourage you to seek further help via your GP or other nutritional specialist, or contact the Eating Disorders Association on 0845 634 1414 or email helpmail@edauk.com.

# Acknowledgements

This book was a lot of fun to write and the wonderful comments from the trial dieters provided enormous encouragement. My books would not reach the publishers without a great team to help me. So a big thank you to Jo Gibbs, who helped sort out the initial applications from everyone who wanted to go on the trial diet, also to Melody Patterson whose job it was to supervise the trial from start to finish, and a fantastic job she did too. Thanks also go to Linda Stevens for the marathon shopping trips where she carefully chose branded products that contained less than four per cent fat so that I could select and compile the diet menus. Special thanks must go to my PA, Louise Cowell, without whom I could not function. Louise co-ordinated everything and made sure that the manuscript was typed on time and that it was complete; also to Dr Andrew Prentice from the Dunn Clinical Nutrition Centre for confirming that the diet was nutritionally sound; to Mary Morris, Training and Development Manager for Rosemary Conley Diet & Fitness Clubs for her most valuable contribution and encouragement in designing particularly effective exercises suitable for inclusion in this book.

My thanks are due also to the many Rosemary Conley Diet & Fitness Clubs members who contributed their favourite recipes. The recipes were tested by a team of pupils at King Edward VII Community College, Coalville, Leicestershire under the careful supervision of Home Economist Lynne Peebles. Lynne and her students ensured that the recipes would be enjoyed by readers of this book.

Particular thanks must go to the trial team recruited by ITV's *This Morning* programme who put the diet to the test and also to all those followers of the first *Flat Stomach Plan* who completed and returned the questionnaire. Their hard work and determination produced the most incredible results and provided the proof that the diet really, really worked.

The unsung hero of any book is the editor. I have worked with Jan Bowmer on all my books since my *Hip and Thigh Diet*. Jan is a dear friend who works incredibly hard to get the job done and done well. Thank you particularly for all your help and hard work with this book, Jan. Also my grateful thanks to Mark Scott and his lovely staff at Stapleford Country House Hotel where I hid myself away in order to complete this book. The magnificent surroundings were most conducive to my concentration on the job in hand, and the fact that I could take along our two dogs to keep me company was greatly appreciated not only by me but particularly by Nikki and Sheba!

Thank you also to Dennis Barker, Art Director at Arrow Books, and to Roger Walker, text designer, for their hard work. This book would not have been possible without this hard-working and professional team. Thank you all so much.

# 1

## So You Want a Flat Stomach?

'I can't believe I've lost 11 inches from my abdomen and nine inches from my waist,' wrote Jacqueline Robson from Fife, after following the Flat Stomach Plan diet for just eight weeks.

Male, female, young or old, everyone would love to have a flatter stomach, and this book will help you achieve just that. But more than that, you will also enjoy significant benefits to your health and vitality – and that's a promise!

You should never write off your tummy by convincing yourself it is simply 'meant to be big', as certainly there's a lot you can do to improve its shape. It doesn't take hours of daily exercise or starvation diets to reduce the fat. What you need is the correct combination of low-fat eating, moderate amounts of aerobic exercise and some strength or toning exercises for the abdominal area. This is the magic formula.

My original Flat Stomach Plan was published at

the end of 1994. It comprised a 28-day diet and fitness programme specifically aimed at reducing the fat on the tummy and was designed in such a way as to encourage even the most undisciplined of dieters.

A team of one thousand volunteers tested the diet and exercises prior to publication. The trial was run 'blind' so that the volunteers were unaware that the stomach was the target area. Consequently, there was no 'encouragement' for dieters to emphasise benefits to specific body areas. You can read more about the trial and its findings in Chapter 2.

The book was an instant number one bestseller and helped hundreds of thousands of people to shed their unwanted inches and rediscover their waistlines. A questionnaire was included in the book so that dieters could report back to me with their progress. The results were fantastic, with a staggering 88 per cent claiming that they were more successful on this diet than any other they had tried before.

Angela Langley from Middlesex wrote: 'I was actually amazed how quickly my weight and measurements changed. I'm now into my 25th week and have lost an unbelievable 4st 7lb.' Norma Ashton from Manchester lost four inches off her waist and five and a half inches off her abdomen. She wrote: 'I feel much better in my health and confidence. My cholesterol level has lowered and my stomach is flat again!'

Now this new Complete Flat Stomach Plan offers you the widest-ever choice of low-fat meals, including an extensive selection of 'instant' branded products for those who are in a hurry or want to snack on something hot in their lunch break, plus loads of motivation to keep you going. It also includes the ultimate exercise plan to help you to a flatter stomach, plus advice on keeping your tummy flat for good. Throughout the book you can read the encouraging comments from those who have already followed the programme and proved that it really does work. Every quote and statistic is accurately reported and carefully filed at my office.

Before we go further, I must stress that I am not suggesting you can spot-reduce through diet or exercise. However, there's no doubt that eating low-fat food within a calorie-controlled diet does *effectively* and *dramatically* reduce the level of adipose tissue (that's fat) stored on the body. My own extensive research has confirmed that by combining low-fat eating with regular aerobic exercise, you *can* lose fat from those stubborn areas, particularly the stomach, hips and thighs.

Followers of my diet and fitness books (and videos) will know that I discovered by accident that low-fat eating leads to a leaner body. In 1986, I was forced on to a low-fat way of eating in order to avoid surgery for gallstones. Having previously 'eaten fat for Britain', this change in eating habits had a dramatic effect on my body. I lost only six pounds in weight, going from 8st 7lb to 8st 1lb, but the transformation in my shape was astonishing. I appeared to have lost those six pounds solely from my hips and thighs.

Realising that I had made an amazing discovery, I designed a low-fat diet plan and put it to the test with a team of volunteers. One hundred and twenty enthusiastic dieters completed the trial and returned their questionnaires. The results were incredible. Everyone lost weight and inches *and* confirmed my own findings – *that low-fat eating really does lead to a significant reduction in the body's fat stores, particularly from those hard-to-slim areas.*

If you follow a low-fat diet you will reduce the fat from the 'fattest' areas of your body. So, if you are pear-shaped, as I am, you will lose fat mainly around your hips and thighs. If you're apple-shaped you'll lose it most from your waist and abdomen, and if you're heart-shaped you will lose it most from your upper body. This may sound obvious, but with most other weight-reducing diets that restrict the calories but not the fat, these areas are the last to reduce. If we eat fat we will store it as fat on our bodies, and we will store it in the specific areas that determine our body shape.

I am not suggesting that we can change our basic body shape, because we can't. But we *can* dramatically improve it. I went from the shape of a Williams pear to a Conference pear – still a pear shape but a narrower one – and ended up a whole dress size smaller below the waist!

## Dispelling a few myths

Many people believe that they can achieve a flatter stomach by doing hundreds of sit-ups every day. However, although sit-ups will *strengthen* your

4

tummy muscles so that you can pull them in more easily, they won't reduce the fat.

Another misconception is that you can turn fat into muscle through exercise – that there's some miraculous biochemical reaction within the body that transforms the fat into lean muscle tissue. This is not so. You can no more turn fat into muscle than you can turn a cat into a dog – they are completely different.

## What will work

The only way to achieve a flatter stomach is to literally burn away the fat that sits contentedly on our tums. This way, the fat disappears in the same way that a log disappears when we burn it in the fire grate. There are two ways we can achieve this: through aerobic exercise and through low-fat, calorie-controlled eating. If we combine the two – bingo! And the good news is that it is easier than you may think.

Just as a car needs fuel to enable it to run, our body also needs fuel in the form of calories to enable it to function and allow us to accomplish our day-to-day tasks. Even when we are sleeping, our bodies need fuel to carry out lots of bodily functions such as tissue-repairing and renewing, digestion, breathing, pumping blood around the body, and a million and one other things. As soon as we step out of bed in the morning, we start using more fuel than we did when we were resting and just 'ticking over'.

The energy content of food is measured in calories. The average daily calorie requirement for women is around 2,200, while men need between 2,500 and 3,500, depending on their activity level. If we want to lose weight, the calorie intake should be reduced to between 1,400 and 1,500 per day for women and between 1,700 and 2,200 for men. Once we cut down on the calories, the body calls upon its 'in-house' fat stores to make up the shortfall – in the same way that we might top up the petrol tank in the car using petrol from the spare can in the boot.

This simple principle forms the basis of all weight-reducing diets. If we eat too many calories we *gain* weight and we store the excess of fat. It's like filling lots of spare petrol cans with fuel that is not needed at present. As far as our bodies are concerned, that extra fuel is stored as fat in 'safe deposit' boxes (fat cells) on our tummies, hips, thighs or chest, depend-ing on our specific body shape. Of course, we will store fat in other areas too, but the fat is more readily stored in our 'problem' areas, where we have a greater number of fat cells. That's why they become problem areas in the first place!

Anyone can lose weight if they eat fewer calories than their body needs. That is a fact. But we now know that we can actually maximise fat loss by eating a low-fat diet and undertaking regular aerobic exercise. However, it's important to understand that weight loss is not as important as inch loss. When we lose inches, it's a sure sign that the fat is disappearing and, after all, that's our goal.

When I devise a diet, I do the calorie counting for you. So you don't have to worry about that. Attempt-ing to count every calorie and then realising that you have exceeded your calorie allowance for the day is the most likely cause of anyone 'throwing in the towel' and abandoning the diet. I tell you what you can eat, but your success is down to you. You have to take the decision to stick to the diet and not to cheat. Your calorie consumption may vary slightly according to which menus you select, but such variations will almost certainly average out over a week or so.

The fat content of each meal included in this Complete Flat Stomach Plan diet has been carefully considered to ensure that you eat an adequate amount of fat to stay healthy yet in sufficiently small quantities to enable you to maximise your weight and inch loss. If you eat what I tell you, you will lose weight and inches, and that's a guarantee.

Recent clinical research has proved that the body is very inefficient at utilising fat in the diet as an energy source and, instead, prefers to use carbohydrate for fuel. Ounce for ounce, carbohydrate contains less than half the calories of fat, so it is clear to see that fat is bad news for the dieter. Too much fat in the diet can also be harmful to health, and I have had many reports from both my trial team and others who have followed my low-fat diets that their health has subsequently improved.

Of course, diets come in all styles and disguises, but beware of those which promise unrealistic weight losses and that recommend a very low calorie intake of, say, less than 1,000 calories a day. If we feed the body too few calories, it switches over to 'emergency mode' and begins burning protein (muscle tissue) for fuel instead of using its fat stores. Any food that is eaten is then rapidly converted into fat and stored. This is Nature's way of protecting us from starving to death. On my low-fat diets, however, you are allowed lots of food so that neither you nor your body is deprived. You won't feel as if you are 'dieting' – you'll just be eating healthily.

The World Health Organisation recommends that fat should form no more than one third of our total daily calorie intake. In real terms, this equates to about 70 grams of fat per day for the average woman whose total calorie requirement would be about 2,200 per day. *This means a woman who is not trying to lose weight but who is just eating to be healthy.* To lose weight we need to eat significantly less fat than that, although I would not recommend that anyone eats less than 25 grams per day.

Just as I actively discourage calorie counting, I also discourage the counting of fat grams. Instead, we should build up a knowledge of which foods are low in fat and which should be avoided, and this automatic gauging system should govern the foods we buy and eat in years to come.

All *you* need to do is follow the advice contained in the following pages, and your waistline will become smaller, your tummy flatter, your hips and thighs narrower, and your energy levels and sense of wellbeing will increase dramatically. Try it for a month, and just watch the transformation. You'll never want to go back to eating high fat again.

# 2
# Tried and Tested

After receiving so many requests from the general public to write a book that would help people to achieve a flatter stomach, two years ago I set about the task. I knew that a low-fat diet could help reduce the fat on the hips and thighs of pear-shaped people, so there was no reason why it shouldn't reduce the fat on the tummies of those who were apple-shaped. I decided that if I devised a new selection of low-fat menus that offered plenty to eat so that no one would feel deprived and combined it with some aerobic exercise to burn the fat along with some toning exercises to strengthen the abdomen, then it had to work. However, as with my Hip and Thigh Diet, I wanted to put it to the test to ensure that it did.

As the diet and fitness expert on ITV's *This Morning* programme with Judy Finnigan and Richard Madeley, I had the perfect opportunity to ask for volunteers from the public. So we announced on air that I was looking for 250 volunteers to try out a new diet and invited viewers to write in and apply. Within just a few days we were inundated, having received no less than 24,000 applications! Unfortunately, it was not possible to respond to them all, so we selected one thousand volunteers from those people we could identify as being apple-shaped.

Where possible, we also gave preference to people who were existing members of my diet and fitness clubs so that we could achieve a more accurate record of actual fat loss. Anyone who commences a diet for the first time will often lose a significant amount of weight in the first week due to a reduction in fluid levels within the body as a result of the change in food consumed. By inviting existing members of my clubs, we would therefore avoid this artificial weight loss and arrive at a really genuine result.

We also chose people who had only a moderate amount of weight to lose in preference to those who were clinically obese (i.e. weighing more than twice their recommended weight) as, again, we wanted to achieve a wholly realistic average. Obviously, someone who was grossly overweight would achieve a much greater weight loss which would give an artificial swing to the final results.

My greatest sadness was that we could not include all 24,000 volunteers. I hope they went on to try the Flat Stomach Plan when it was published and found that it worked for them.

The members of the trial team were sent a pack which included the trial diet (unnamed) and a short programme of exercise. They were asked to eat three meals a day from the menu choices given and recommended to do 15 minutes of aerobic exercise each day. In addition they were asked to do a selection of toning exercises as often as possible each week.

We also supplied them with an extensive questionnaire, which they were asked to complete and return after four weeks on the diet. Remember, they had no idea which part of the body we were targeting.

These were the results:

71.3 per cent said they *lost most inches from their waist and abdomen.*

88.7 per cent said that they had been more successful on this diet than on any other diet they had tried before.

98.4 per cent lost both weight and inches.

75 per cent said they were surprised by their inch losses.

80 per cent enjoyed better health.

95 per cent said they enjoyed the diet.

Over the four-week period, the average loss of those who had followed the diet moderately strictly (54 per cent) was a very satisfactory 8.4lb. But for the 44 per cent who stuck to it very strictly, the reward was an excellent 10.2lb loss. All the experts agree that a weight loss of around two pounds per week is ideal because this means that the weight lost will consist mostly of fat.

Thirty-two per cent of the trial dieters noticed a reduction in their cellulite which was an added bonus. When asked if they had any problems with constipation, 83 per cent said that they either had no problems or had noticed an improvement in previous symptoms.

I asked if my dieters had binged at all during the diet. Seventy-six per cent said they had not binged at all.

Four per cent said this was the first diet they had tried, and 40 per cent said they had dieted occasionally before. Fifty-six per cent said they had been on more diets than they cared to remember but that they had been more successful on this diet than on any other diet.

When we make dramatic changes in our eating habits, it is always interesting to note any changes that may occur in our bodies. With this in mind, I asked my dieters if they had experienced any change in the condition of their hair, skin and fingernails. Twenty-two per cent had noticed an improvement in the condition of their hair, while 76 per cent said there was no change. Under two per cent said the condition of their hair had deteriorated.

Thirty-four per cent reported an improvement in the condition of their skin, while six per cent said there was no change. Only four per cent said their skin had deteriorated.

Thirty per cent of dieters noticed an improvement in the condition of their nails, while 66 per cent said that their nails had remained the same. Four per cent said their nails had deteriorated. These statistics were particularly encouraging because, in most cases, the condition of the hair, skin and nails had not deteriorated while some people had noticed a positive improvement. The number of people who noticed a deterioration was negligible and, in any case, this could have been caused by lifestyle changes unconnected to the diet.

Almost all the dieters had done some aerobic and toning exercise and the majority reported that their fitness level had improved.

When asked if they had been more successful on this diet than on previous diets, those who answered yes were asked to stipulate why by choosing from a list of multi-choice answers. The reasons given were that this diet was easier to follow; it involved no calorie counting; it offered more freedom of choice; it was quite different from any other diet they had tried before; they could have a drink without feeling guilty; they could eat so much more than on most other diets; and perhaps, most important of all, they had greater willpower because they were part of a trial team.

There is no doubt that this last reason was extremely significant, because motivation is the key to success. I have therefore devoted an entire chapter to this (see Chapter 4).

The biggest weight loss was achieved by Sally Green from Leicestershire who went from 14st 8lb to 12st 3lb in four weeks. Sally continued on the diet and after eight weeks had reduced her weight by a total of 42 pounds. Sally's incredible rate of weight loss was no doubt enhanced by the fact that she was a rock 'n' roll dancer in her spare time. She wrote: 'I go rock 'n' roll dancing and have improved my timing as I now have not so much bulk to pull around as I twirl!' Rock on, Sally.

Hilary Dearden of Birmingham summed up her results: 'I cannot thank you enough for showing me a new Hilary who doesn't get tired after running for a bus, who doesn't fall asleep every time she gets in from work and who finally has the courage to try on wedding dresses for the big day.

'PS When I started the diet I weighed more than my sister who was eight months pregnant at the time! It is now my turn to borrow her clothes while mine are being used to supplement her maternity clothes!'

Another stunning success story was Mrs Dora Lilley from Hampshire. Dora lost 21 pounds in the first four weeks and a staggering 11 inches from her waist. She stayed with the diet and lost a further 13 pounds in the next four weeks and two more inches off her waistline, making a total loss of 13 inches from her waist. Dora wrote: 'My husband was so impressed that he has now started the diet, and my children brought me a bouquet of flowers. I do not suffer pain in my ankles and feet any more and my feet do not swell.'

Angela Wait, who attends a Rosemary Conley class in Sheffield, had already lost two stone and 36 inches in the previous seven months on the Hip and Thigh Diet. On her application form she stated that she still had some excess weight to lose which had been hanging around since the birth of her children. When she started the trial diet she weighed only 10st 4½lb, which was not excessive for her 5ft 8in height. After four weeks she lost six and a half pounds and a remarkable five and a half inches from around her tummy.

Angela wrote: 'I must say I am *very* pleased with the weight and inch loss in the past four weeks, especially from my stomach. After having two babies, this is a problem area. I am quite amazed – my abdomen started at 40 inches and after four weeks is now 34½ inches.'

After four more weeks Angela lost a further two pounds to bring her down to a very trim 9st 10lb and a significantly flatter stomach, which was now seven inches smaller than when she had started the trial. She commented: 'I am amazed at how many inches I lost from my abdomen. I did not follow the diet as strictly in the last four weeks, but I am still pleased – no, delighted – with the results.'

Some of the other inch losses were also quite astonishing. Norma Carter from Devon lost eight pounds in the first four weeks and an incredible seven inches from her abdomen.

Susan Chalmers from Northern Ireland lost a remarkable 1st 4lb in the first four weeks of the plan and decided to stick with it. After eight weeks Susan had lost an amazing 28 pounds, plus five inches from her tummy and six inches from her waist. Before starting the trial, dieters had been asked to sign an agreement in which they promised not to show the plan to anyone or make a photocopy of it. Susan wrote: 'My best friends offered me money to learn my dietary secrets.'

She went on to say: 'I feel much less bulky and my joints don't ache so much. Losing so much inside such a short amount of time has given me a real boost mentally.'

Nicole Aries from Woking lost 14 pounds in the first four weeks and a further nine pounds in the second four weeks. She wrote: 'The trial may be over, but I'm sticking to this!'

If at any time you need further inspiration or convincing that the diet really does work, please turn to Chapter 10. This chapter contains additional comments and quotes both from trial dieters and also from those who followed the diet and exercise plan from the Flat Stomach Plan book.

Numerous people also reported significant benefits to their general health, with some experiencing improvements to long-standing medical conditions. A selection of their comments is included in Chapter 11.

# 3
# The Television Trial Team

Out of the thousand people who took part in the diet trial, we selected eight who allowed us to film their progress for the *This Morning* television programme. The team of eight formed a cross-section of occupations, lifestyles, ages, weights, with varying histories of success or failure in terms of weight loss. They were invited to my head office at Quorn House where I briefed them on the diet. Each of them was given a diet sheet, together with a questionnaire which they were to complete after four weeks. They were asked to stay on the diet for eight weeks and to monitor their progress carefully. Here's a profile of their experiences.

Lyn and Robert Sanchez from Cheshire volunteered to do the diet together. Lyn was in her mid-thirties and Robert a little older. Neither was very over-weight, but both felt that losing a stone or two would be beneficial to their health. Lyn was tall at 5ft 9in and weighed 12st 2lb at the beginning of the trial, while Robert at 6ft 1in weighed in at 16st 1lb.

After four weeks, they had both lost ten pounds. Robert had lost ten inches overall and Lyn had lost 14 inches. After a further four weeks, Robert had lost an additional eight pounds and now weighed in at 14st 2lb, and Lyn weighed in at a trim 10st 11lb.

At the beginning of the trial Robert admitted that he had a typical male outlook and thought that 'it would just be lettuce leaves and nothing else, but I was pleasantly surprised at the amount of food you could eat and the variety.' At the end of the eight weeks, he said: 'I feel a lot healthier. I find that I can run around for a lot longer than I used to be able to.'

Lyn was also pleased with her results: 'I certainly feel healthier and have a lot more energy. I have found that I have re-educated my shopping trolley. I have learned to prepare food differently. I am absolutely delighted – it has been so easy.'

Robert had experienced no problems with the exercise programme since he exercised already and it just meant building up to a set routine each week. Lyn said that she found the recommended 15 minutes a day of aerobic exercise totally unobtrusive but wanted a more structured plan and therefore went to two classes a week.

When we came to film Lyn and Robert at Ragdale Hall shortly after the end of the eight-week trial, they looked like film stars, having lost 18 pounds and 17 pounds respectively. Their beautifully toned figures and the pounds they had shed made a dramatic difference to their overall appearance. They were an inspiration to us all.

The next member of our TV trial team was Gillian Woodroffe from Liverpool. Gillian had pleaded with us to give her a chance to be part of the trial team. Gillian's husband Dave, a policeman, was not 'officially' included in the trial team but ultimately became part of it as he joined Gillian on the diet. Fortunately, we had inadvertently filmed him at home, so we were able to show the viewers the dramatic transformation that occurred.

At the start of the trial, Gillian weighed in at 12st 9lb, which was a couple of stone overweight for her 5ft 9in height. She had dieted lots of times before and would usually lose a stone when she tried hard, but when she got bored she would put it back on again. At her heaviest, she had weighed 13st 7lb.

After four weeks on the trial, Gillian had lost 11 pounds and, after eight weeks, a total of 25 pounds. Much to our amazement, husband Dave had lost 33 pounds. He had previously weighed in at 16st 3lb and was now down to 13st 12lb. By the time we came to film them at the end of the trial, Dave had lost 40lb in total and eight inches off his stomach. 'I was really surprised how quickly it came off,' he said. 'I found the diet very filling. The amounts that you were allowed were quite substantial and there was more than enough to eat.'

He admitted that he had gone on the diet to support Gillian. 'I knew she had to stick to the diet, so I thought that with me joining in it would give her more support,' he said. 'Apart from that, if I didn't eat what she was eating I would have starved!'

Gillian was delighted with her weight loss. 'I can't believe it. I have never successfully stuck to a diet for this long. It is absolutely great and I feel brilliant,' she said. She admitted that, during the trial, people had noticed Dave's weight loss more than her own. However, she had found it easier to stick to the diet because of Dave's involvement.

There is no doubt that if you can find someone to join in the diet with you, then your chances of success are infinitely greater. When Gillian and Dave came into the television studio to enjoy a make-over live on air, they looked fabulous in their trendy new outfits and the transformation was astonishing.

Another volunteer couple was Shirley and Ian Rockliffe, both of whom were in their mid-twenties. They had two young children – a 22-month-old little girl and Adam, who was just four months old. Shirley was 5ft 4in tall and weighed in at 10st 3lb, while Ian was 5ft 11in and weighed in at 13st 6lb.

Baby Adam had suffered badly with colic and, consequently, Shirley admitted that this left her with little time to prepare proper meals. During the day she had tended to eat things that were easy to open. In the evening, she and Ian would sit down to meals – usually something with chips – and Ian would often pop out to the local shop afterwards for cakes and chocolates. Shirley had a wardrobe full of clothes that she couldn't wear because the buttons were bursting open or the zips wouldn't do up. She had bought a special suit for Adam's christening but was now unable to fasten it. As she was going to be a godmother in a few months' time, she was determined to slim down so that she could wear the suit.

After four weeks on the diet, Shirley had lost 11 pounds and Ian had lost a stone. Eight weeks later, Shirley had lost a total of 1st 3lb and Ian 1st 6lb. By the time we saw Shirley at the end of the trial, she proudly announced that she now ate only three meals a day and had stopped eating chocolate. For the camera, she was able to fit into the skirt of the smart new suit she planned to wear for the christening and, what's more, there were inches to spare.

Shirley was delighted with her new figure: 'I can't believe how flat my stomach is. After I had my first baby, my stomach was never as flat as this,' she said. When we met up later, she told me: 'I got into my suit, but the joke is that, by the time of the christening, the suit was too big!'

Joan Weinman from Manchester was selected for the TV trial because she admitted that being part of a trial team would be more likely to inspire her into action. She felt sufficiently committed that she wouldn't let us down and therefore would benefit by not letting herself down either. Joan admitted that she had always had a weight problem, even when she was at school, and at 5ft 4in she weighed in at 13 stone – the heaviest she had ever been. Much to her surprise, Joan lost ten pounds during the first four weeks, despite the fact she had a slow metabolic rate because of her frequent attempts at dieting.

When we first interviewed her, she said: 'I feel that as I have got older my metabolism has obviously slowed down. It just isn't like it used to be. I am finding it harder and harder to lose weight. When I am depressed I look for sweet foods. I suppose it is comfort eating and I tend to do secret eating. I wait for my husband to take a bath and then I pinch a biscuit, but I pretend to myself that I haven't eaten it. I just feel that the whole world is looking at me, saying, "Oh isn't she fat!" And "Look at her." I look at these slim people – not necessarily young people – and I am envious.'

Over the eight-week period Joan lost a stone and we thought it would be interesting to take her along to Chester College to undergo some tests to check whether Joan had indeed a slow metabolic rate. Chester College has an exceptionally well-fitted laboratory for testing metabolism and other physiological facts. Dr Kevin Sykes, head of the physiology department, did some tests on Joan.

First, he attached Joan to a metabolic measuring machine which was able to tell us how much oxygen her body required just to stand there and do nothing. We learned that Joan needed about 1,500 to 1,600 calories per day just to keep her body ticking over.

Next, Dr Sykes got Joan to walk quite gently on a treadmill. The intensity was slowly increased and Joan had to breathe into a special piece of apparatus so that we could identify at which point the energy source that Joan was using was in fact fat. Dr Sykes told us that Joan's resting metabolic rate, while slightly on the low side, was certainly within the normal range. Now that he had put her into some gentle exercise she was burning a lot more calories than when she was just standing at rest.

For the first ten minutes or so her body was using predominantly carbohydrates as its source of energy. But once Joan had been going for about 15 minutes her body was starting to switch more towards fat as its energy source and burning up to five calories a minute.

Dr Sykes explained that, although five calories a minute might seem a small amount, if such exercise was done on a regular basis then, clearly, Joan would not be burning calories just during exercise, but she would also continue to do so afterwards. Not only that, but her body would become more efficient at burning fat. This was heartening news for Joan who resolved to become more active in her day-to-day life.

There are a number of reasons why some people find it more difficult to lose weight than others. When we gain weight, the fat cells swell up and reach their maximum capacity and so the body makes more fat cells. Therefore, the more weight you gain, the easier it is for your body to create new fat cells. This is one reason why it's important to attempt to keep your weight under control.

Our next stop was nutritionist Penny Hunking. I asked Penny what other factors might affect some people's ability to lose weight.

Penny explained that, there is an enzyme known as lipoprotein lipase – or LPL for short – which is responsible for putting fat into fat cells. When people go on a crash diet, this lipoprotein lipase increases in quantity and, as a result, they become very efficient fat-storers and gain weight easily.

One further factor to be taken into account is the 'set point' theory, which states that your body is happy at a certain weight – even if you're not! It is very difficult to shift your body away from this, but it is thought that exercise may be able to lower this set point.

Joan was reassured by all this information. She accepted that because she had always been over-weight, even as a child, she would never become very slim simply because of the number of fat cells in her body. Secondly, she was now fully aware that any amount of exercise would help her weight-loss campaign. She was relieved to know that she hadn't in fact got a particularly slow metabolic rate and therefore wasn't fighting a losing battle.

I was confident that Joan would keep off the stone she had lost during the trial and that she would succeed in losing even more weight on her new regime.

The next member of our trial team was Janina Stevens from Manchester. Janina was in her mid-thirties and had recently been made redundant. She hoped that losing weight would give her the confidence she needed to clinch that interview and get a new job.

Janina explained that she had put on weight gradually over the years, probably since starting university. Also, her mother had died recently and that had knocked her for six. She believes she put on a lot of weight at that time, as a kind of emotional crutch.

We called on the expertise on Dr Raj Persaud, the psychologist on the *This Morning* programme. I asked Raj why it was that our weight was so important to the way we felt about ourselves.

Raj explained that when researchers asked men what made them feel valued and gave them good self-esteem, it seems that men tend to place importance on their job and how much they earn. For women, however, even those with successful careers, it always seems to come back to the way they look, and that relates to how much they weigh.

Raj felt that there was a lot of pressure for women to be very slim. Many women who come to his surgery and who are trying to lose weight are unrealistic and tend to pick a target weight that is way too low – often 10–15 per cent lower than the weight for which they should really be aiming. The point to remember is that you should aim for a weight that you are going to be able to achieve for the rest of your life.

It is also important to be in the right frame of mind when you start a diet. Raj stressed that any diet that is started with the idea of your hating yourself and being negative about yourself is likely to end in disaster.

One of the overwhelming facts that came through from the trial dieters was that their self-esteem and confidence had absolutely rocketed after they had lost weight. Raj confirmed that most women find that, once they lose a bit of weight, their self-esteem and confidence increases, and this is partly because they now feel better about the way they look and they feel able to be more assertive in their relationships.

At the end of eight weeks, Janina had lost 14 pounds and was brimming with confidence. Delighted, she said: 'Before, my tummy used to be the same measurement as my bust. Now that I have lost 6½ inches off my tummy, you can really see a difference.'

The last member of the trial team was Vivien Molloy from Liverpool. Vivien was in her late twenties and weighed in at 12st 10lb which was too heavy for her 5ft 4in height. She had tried every diet that was going – Weight Watchers, Slimfast, the Cambridge Diet. she had even tried acupuncture and slimming tablets. You name it – she'd tried it! Vivien admitted to being a yo-yo dieter and a binger all her life.

Vivien explained:

'I suppose you could say I am one of those comfort eaters. I eat when I am bored. It is just something to do. My husband is in the TA [territorial army] and he is away two weekends each month. During the day, I'm on the go all the time since I have two little boys. But as soon as they go to bed, I get so fed up and lonely, I have a bottle of wine and then maybe a packet of crisps. And then I think, they were nice, I'll have another packet – and so it goes on. I can be good. I can go for days and days when I stick rigidly to a diet, and then maybe I might have one sweet, but to me it is just like a trigger food. Once I've had a taste of it, I want more.

I asked Raj Persaud why one sneak treat would lead to a binge. Raj replied that if people made a careful note of the times they binged, they would notice that they tend to binge at set times of the day, which usually means that it is linked to a particular emotion. It might be boredom, loneliness, anger or depression. In effect, you are experiencing a negative emotion and you're looking for comfort from that emotion.

One of the things that emerged from the trial was the fact that once the dieters were in the routine of having three meals a day, they found that their inclination to binge was greatly reduced.

Raj said that bingeing was part of a cycle that people get into when they go on extreme diets. Because they are on an extreme diet they feel hungry, so they break their resolve and have a binge. Then, because they've had a binge, they feel guilty and that leads to another period of extreme dieting, and that cycle eventually leads to very chaotic eating behaviour.

He stressed that successful slimming was not just about going on a diet for a couple of weeks. If you want to change your weight or your body shape, it involves changing your whole life. You can't just tinker with one small part of the system, such as eating or exercise. You have to think about every aspect of your life and change the way you think about yourself.

After eight weeks on the trial diet, Vivien lost a total of 18 inches and 22 pounds. She commented: 'I found that on the actual diet you could eat enough and I didn't want to binge, whereas, before, I would starve myself all day and I would be starving by the end of the night and eat loads. With this diet, it doesn't work like that at all.'

I asked Vivien how she coped when her husband was away. Vivien replied: 'This time I told myself that I will do my exercise video, then I'll go and have my bubble bath. I'll have my glass of wine which I'm allowed and save my banana from my main meal to eat later. I felt more in control doing it that way, and I would go to bed happy.'

I had to smile when Vivien told me: 'I can't believe the difference it's made. I used to wear my coat all the time, even in summer. I'd be roasting hot but I wouldn't take it off. Now I can go out all the time without my coat on. I'm freezing cold going to the school to pick up the children, but I don't care!'

All our trial dieters proved to be absolute stars and a delight to work with. During the filming we visited several locations – Chester College, Ragdale Hall and Chester Zoo, where we met Sheba the four-ton elephant who represented the total amount of weight lost by the entire trial team. Ros Peters, the producer from Granada, did a superb job in designing the series so that we were able to convey a meaningful, motivational and inspirational message to the viewers.

# Trial team round-up

Prior to this book going to press, we rang the members of the TV trial team to see how they were faring. These were the results.

### Lyn and Robert Sanchez

Both maintained their weight loss well and easily. However, Lyn is now 20 weeks pregnant and is only gaining weight at a steady and sensible rate. She is determined that she will *not* gain the 4½ stone that she gained during her last pregnancy and feels confident that she will quickly regain her figure after the birth.

Lyn and Robert continue to follow the basic principles of healthy, low-fat eating and feel that they now definitely eat a more sensible diet than they ever did before.

### Gillian and David Woodroffe

Both have maintained their weight loss with no problems.

### Shirley and Ian Rockliffe

Both have maintained their weight loss with no problems.

### Joan Weinman

Joan has not regained any weight, despite suffering a fairly serious illness which meant she was unable to exercise for many weeks. Joan's husband has also had a heart problem, so they both now eat a healthy, low-fat diet.

### Vivien Molloy

Unfortunately, Vivien has had a few personal problems and has regained some of her weight. However, she has resolved to try and lose it again as she was so delighted with her previous success.

# 4

# How Badly Do You Want a Flat Stomach?

If someone offered you £50,000 if you were able to achieve a flat stomach, do you think you could do it? Of course you could. Why? Because the reward would be great enough to inspire you to make the effort and put into practice all that was needed to achieve that goal. You would want to achieve it so badly that you wouldn't let anything get in your way and allow you to stray off course.

This book contains all the information you need to achieve a flat stomach. It's up to you to do the rest. As I explained earlier, if you have a big stomach, it's because you are storing fat in that area by eating more food than your body needs as fuel. To achieve a flatter stomach you need to burn away the fat by increasing your level of physical activity, and you need to reduce your food intake so that your body calls upon its reserves of fat to make up the shortfall.

Eating a low-fat diet will ensure that you do not replenish those fat stores. In addition, if you do some specific abdominal exercises you can improve the strength and muscle tone around your middle. By combining all these factors you will definitely achieve a significantly flatter stomach.

However, having acquired all the 'know-how' you now have to put it into practice. You need to make some definite plans when you go shopping at the supermarket. You will have to make some changes when you prepare food in the kitchen. You will have to make time in your busy lifestyle to do the exercises, and you will need a good dose of willpower to make the right choices when you dine out.

There's one further vital ingredient that you will need and that is a positive attitude towards your diet and fitness campaign. This chapter is intended to help you develop a positive mental attitude so that success is inevitable. Whether it be in our work, our hobbies or our family life, there are those people who just drift through their lives. But the ones who have the motivation to succeed are the great achievers. I want to help you become a great achiever as far as your diet and fitness campaign is concerned.

In my original Flat Stomach Plan, which gave a day-by-day diet and exercise plan, I also included a positive thought for each day. The reason for this was to give each day a purpose and to set a task or challenge for the dieter. I know from the letters I received that many readers found these particularly helpful and motivational, so here is some further advice which I hope will inspire you.

## Set yourself a goal

If you want to lose weight, get fit and achieve a flatter stomach you need to have a goal to aim for. In this instance, I'm not talking about losing a set amount of inches from around your waist or being able to get into a size 10 or down to a certain weight. I am talking about a goal that provides a deadline for you to work towards and a reason for losing as much weight as possible by that date.

For instance, athletes have specific sporting events to work towards. This enables them to plan their training programme so that they can achieve their ultimate performance on that particular day. Salesmen, likewise, have targets to reach within a specific period of time and they will work incredibly hard to achieve those targets. The point is that we all work better and achieve more if we have a deadline to meet. Most people have events in their diaries – a wedding, a special celebration, a holiday or a job interview – by which time they want to look their absolute best. If you have no such date in your diary, give yourself a target to reach, say, in two months' time. The target should be realistic – don't expect to lose four stone in two months – but it should provide a sufficiently great challenge so that you have to concentrate your mind and energy to achieve it.

And once you have achieved your goal, it is important that you reward yourself. For many, it may be sufficient reward to be able to look stunning in a new outfit at the wedding or special celebration. If you don't have a specific event to attend, then reward yourself with a trip to a health farm, a meal out with a partner or friend or treat yourself to a new outfit. If you can get someone else to treat you, then so much the better! Tell the rest of the family of your plans and ask them to encourage you along the way. Let them be part of the celebration so that they have a vested interest in your success. You may find that other family members will be happy to join you in your crusade towards a healthier body and that the whole exercise becomes a team effort, one that you all enjoy together.

Once you have reached that first goal date, you need to set another date to provide you with the motivation to stick with your new diet and fitness regime. Even if you have already achieved your target weight, you will need an incentive to encourage you to stay at that weight.

At a recent seminar on the management of obesity, Dr Christopher Fairburn from the Department of Psychiatry at Oxford University explained that the act of losing weight is rewarding but that maintaining the loss is often difficult and unrewarding, which is why so many fail. He stressed that it was vital to continue exercising and receive ongoing support if that weight loss is to be maintained. We all need encouragement, and this is one of the great benefits for those who attend a Rosemary Conley Diet & Fitness Club. Members can still enjoy the ongoing benefit of regular exercise at the classes once they have achieved their goal weight. Having a reason to attend other than just to be weighed serves a dual purpose. The ladies work out and keep their weight in check. This is why our success rate in weight maintenance is so high compared with other weight-loss systems.

## Stop making excuses

There will never be a week or a month when there isn't a birthday, a special meal out, or a million and one other reasons why this isn't a good time to start a diet. We need to accept that these times of temptation form part of everyday life. It is essential that we stop making excuses – and I think I've heard them all – and really get on with the job in hand. If you want a flat stomach and you want to lose weight and get fit, you can. Only *you* can do it, and you have to want to do it badly enough. So stop making excuses and get on with it.

## Be realistic

Just as we cannot change our height or our genes, neither can we change our bone structure, or basic physiological shape. Accepting these basic criteria, we can still do one heck of a lot to improve our appearance. It's unrealistic to imagine that we can look like a top model at the end of it. That doesn't mean to say that we can't look stunning, but we are all unique individuals. Never underestimate how much better we can look when we lose those unwanted pounds. Healthy eating and regular exercise can make us glow with health, tone us up as we slim down and give us a greater sense of wellbeing.

Lots of successful slimmers take the big step to change their image: they have a new hairstyle, start dressing more adventurously and find an inner confidence they never knew they possessed. The compliments flow, their self-esteem rises and they achieve so much more in their lives. We don't have to look like a film star to be happy and successful. We just need to be happy with ourselves.

## Record your progress

It is so easy to forget what we look like at our fattest, how big we actually were in terms of inches and what it actually felt like. Before you start this Complete Flat Stomach Plan, first take a couple of photographs of yourself – a front and side view. You do not need to show these to anyone, at least not until you are slim. Next, find yourself a pair of tight-fitting trousers or a skirt and set this aside as your measuring garment. Keep trying on this garment every few days so that you have tangible proof of how much weight and how many inches you are actually losing.

Make a note of your various measurements before you commence the plan. Take the largest measurement around your bust, the smallest around your waist, the largest measurement around your hips, the measurement around your widest part, the largest measurement around the tops of your thighs and/or backside. Measure each thigh at the fattest part, and measure the narrowest part above each knee. Measure around the fattest part of each arm. Record all these measurements on the chart on page 336.

Measure yourself at the same time each week. Ideally ask someone to help you – if your partner can be encouraged to measure you, they will be able to witness your progress and encourage you as those inches disappear. It really is helpful to get your partner involved in your weight-loss campaign.

Weigh yourself at the same time each week. Use the same scales and wear the same clothes – or preferably none. It's a good idea to draw up a graph for each stone you lose. To do this, put the number of weeks along the top, and the number of pounds (from 1–14) down the side. Each week, place a dot in the appropriate spot to mark the number of pounds you have lost. By connecting the dots as you go along you will be able to see your line of progress, and this will encourage you to continue (see sample graph, page 338). Draw up a new graph for each further stone you want to lose. If you wish, you could also make a separate graph to record your inch losses.

Another tip is to keep a carrier bag to hand by the scales and, after each weighing session, to place an item equivalent to the weight you have lost (e.g. a pound bag of sugar) in the bag. If ever you doubt your progress, you can lift up the bag and instantly feel how much weight you have lost. Of course, if you gain weight at any stage, then you will have to remove an item. This suggestion came from one of my franchisees. She asked each of her members to bring to class a bag of food representing their weight loss. The food collected was then taken over to Bosnia in a container lorry by the husband of one of the members. Apart from the fact that this was a great scheme, the members had not appreciated fully the weight they had lost until they carried in their heavy loads. It is so easy for us to forget our progress and we need a constant reminder of our achievements.

## Develop the habit of enthusiasm

There are two ways we can look at our diet and fitness campaign. We can moan about the foods we can't eat and grumble about the prospect of exercise, but if we adopt this attitude, we achieve nothing. It is much better to be enthusiastic and focus on the many benefits you will be enjoying within days of starting your campaign.

Make a note in your diary of all the good things you feel about yourself. Day one might read: 'It's great to go to bed without feeling bloated. I don't feel hungry and I enjoyed my exercise.' On day two you might write: 'I feel slimmer and more energetic. I found the exercise easier today.' You get my drift – look for the good in everything. As your whole attitude towards yourself and your body changes, your self-esteem will increase. It is quite incredible how a positive attitude has a beneficial effect on everyone around us. This fact came through so strongly from the questionnaires that I received from the trial dieters. The feeling of 'I'm succeeding and I am so happy about it' improved everyone's self-esteem and sense of achievement. Your enthusiasm will, in turn, also cause others to be encouraging and complimentary towards your progress, which will see you through even the toughest times.

## Picture yourself succeeding

Picture yourself wearing that beautiful dress you have had in your wardrobe for years but haven't been able to get into. Imagine yourself on the beach in a bikini, feeling proud of your body. Visualise yourself standing tall and slim, full of confidence, as you hold your own at a cocktail party. Picture yourself feeling really healthy and fit with lots of energy and not flagging by the end of the day. If you can really take these thoughts into your mind they will become part of the overall picture and you will be able to translate them into reality. The things you are picturing must be exciting enough for you to want to achieve them.

## Remove temptation

If you are to succeed in your healthy eating plan it is essential that you remove temptation away from your kitchen and from your place of work. You cannot be expected to walk past the biscuit tin when it's brimming full of chocolate digestives and expect your willpower to be strong at all times. If you must have some sweet or high-fat foods in the house, keep them stored away in a place that's difficult to reach or under lock and key. If the food isn't there, you won't miss it, but if it is staring you in the face you will find it very difficult to resist. Similarly, store any hard cheese that you may have bought for the rest of the family in the fridge in a non-see-through container so that it isn't visible each time you open the door. Keep any foods that might tempt you out of sight.

## Learn to cope with the difficult times

No matter how determined and conscientious you may be, there will be occasions when your willpower weakens and your determination begins to flag. It may be that someone has upset you, it may be the time of the month, or you may simply feel fed up. Whatever it is, if you do have a minor indiscretion – or even a major one – do not feel that all is lost. Go back on the diet and, soon, whatever you overate will get used up and burned away so that the damage will be minimal. Having the odd biscuit or the odd chocolate is not going to cause you to regain the pounds or stones that you have lost. Eating the whole packet of biscuits or the whole box of chocolates, however, will certainly cause some 'serious' damage, so don't say to yourself: 'Well, I have had one biscuit so I might as well finish off the packet.' You will be really glad you didn't.

Remember, it's your desire to be slim, fit and healthy, not just your ability to do so, that will determine your success. If that desire goes, temptation will creep in and take over. Remember how miserable you felt when you were overweight. Please don't ever return there.

So, by the time you have read this book, you will

know how to achieve a flatter stomach and healthier body, you will know how to get fit and you will have found a reason for wanting to do it badly enough. Keep concentrating on those goals by setting yourself targets and rewarding yourself when you achieve them, and make a note of good things that happen to you from now on. Keep a scrapbook of your successes. Fill it with photographs of yourself as you lose each stone and look back to see how much you have slimmed down. Take a photograph each time you do something new that you wouldn't have done when you were overweight. Make a note of any compliments that people pay you, no matter how small. Record your personal feelings – how you felt more confident with your partner, how you had more energy to go swimming with the children. All these things are worth noting down. Include the date and also the weight you were on that particular day. Look back at this scrapbook on the 'bad' days and use it to motivate you to get back on the straight and narrow.

# 5
# Getting the Most Out of This Plan

## Eating for health

If we want a slim and healthy body, it's not enough just to cut down on the quantities of food we eat, we also need to ensure we eat a variety of foods to obtain a good balance of nutrients from our diet. The five major nutrients are carbohydrate, protein, vitamins, minerals and fat.

**Carbohydrates** are energy-giving foods. Eating carbohydrate is the equivalent of putting petrol in your car. Carbohydrates come in two varieties, complex and simple. Simple carbohydrates, or sugars, contain largely 'empty calories' and very few nutrients. Complex carbohydrates, on the other hand, include starchy foods such as bread, potatoes, cereal, pasta and rice. The body is very efficient at converting complex carbohydrates into energy and therefore the bulk of our diet should be made up of these.

However, I'm not giving you a licence to eat unlimited amounts, because if you do, you'll gain weight – remember the spare cans of petrol in Chapter 1? But it is absolutely fine to have cereal and/or toast for breakfast, a sandwich or jacket potato for lunch and a main evening meal that includes pasta, rice or potatoes. Because you will be eating lots of carbohydrates on the Complete Flat Stomach Plan diet you should have loads of energy. In turn, this will encourage you to be more physically active so that you burn more calories and get slimmer more quickly.

**Proteins** are used by the body for growth and repair, not just during our 'growing' years, but for ever. The body is constantly working at renewing itself to replace worn-out bits, to repair tissue and enable our hair, skin and nails to grow.

Meat, poultry, fish, milk, eggs, yogurt and cheese are all complete sources of protein. Foods such as pulses (that's beans and lentils), grains, nuts and seeds do contain protein, but this protein is 'incomplete'. To form complete proteins, therefore, it is necessary for pulses, grains, nuts or seeds to be eaten together in any combination of two or combined with a complete protein. This is not as complicated as it sounds. For example, you could choose beans on toast (pulse and grain), or a bean salad with a low-fat yogurt (pulse and dairy product), cereal with milk (grain and dairy product) and so on.

Moderate amounts of protein are utilised very efficiently by the body, but too much can be harmful. Moderation is the key.

**Vitamins** are essential for good health and fulfil numerous bodily functions. A varied diet, such as the one in this book, that also includes plenty of fresh foods, should be rich in vitamins. When selecting your menus, try to ensure you eat two pieces of fresh fruit each day in addition to your 150ml (¼ pint) daily fruit juice allowance. Do take the opportunity to fill up on fresh vegetables and salad with your main meal of the day, as these are allowed in unlimited quantities.

**Minerals** are also vital for good health. Calcium and iron are particularly important. We need calcium for strong bones and teeth. On this diet, you are allowed 450ml (¾ pint) skimmed or semi-skimmed milk daily to ensure you receive plenty of calcium. Dairy produce is also a rich source, but do make sure you select low-fat products to minimise the fat content. Other sources include dark green leafy vegetables such as spinach and broccoli, and sardines, salmon and tofu.

Iron is important for maintaining the level of red blood cells within the bloodstream. Iron is found in liver, kidneys and enriched cereal products, so try to eat at least one serving of these foods each week. Egg yolks are also rich in iron, but because these are also high in fat, I recommend that eggs are restricted to two a week for meat-eaters and three a week for vegetarians. Vitamin C enhances the absorption of iron, so ideally try to combine iron and vitamin C in the same meal, for instance a boiled egg with a glass of orange juice.

**Fat** is the last nutrient group and, as far as we are concerned, the one you need worry about least in terms of deficiency. Certainly, we do need a small amount of fat for good health, but it really is only a small amount. It is important to remember that small amounts of fat are to be found in almost every food we eat – even in lettuce leaves! So, providing we eat a balanced diet, even on a low-fat diet we are unlikely to be deficient.

If you are vegetarian, however, you should add a tiny amount of olive oil to your diet – a drop or two is all you need – as you will not be obtaining fat from meat or fish sources. Accordingly, the vegetarian recipes in this book include a small amount of oil.

Remember that all oils contain 100 per cent fat, butter 80 per cent, Flora 70 per cent, and even low-fat spreads can contain as much as 60 per cent fat! However, oily fish such as mackerel, tuna, salmon and sardines are allowed on this diet, as they contain beneficial fat. The oil from these fish is well utilised by the body and complements an otherwise low-fat diet.

# Reading nutrition labels

We are now fortunate that the nutrient content of most food products is displayed on the packaging. This is of tremendous help to anyone who is watching their weight or their health.

As far as weight control is concerned, there are only two details you need to read carefully on the label – the 'energy' value and the 'fat' content. The energy value will be shown in kilojoules or kilocalories – kJ or kcal for short. The 'kcal' figure will tell you the number of calories per 100 grams.

The fat content may be split as follows:

| FAT | 4g |
| of which saturates | 2.5g |
| unsaturates | 1.5g |

This means that within 100 grams of this product there are four grams of fat. The fat is of two types, saturated (mainly animal original) and unsaturated (plant or fish origin). On a low-fat, weight-reducing diet, however, it's irrelevant where the fat comes from, so you can ignore the finer detail. All you need to know is the total fat content. As a general rule, when selecting foods in the supermarket, choose only those foods that contain four grams – or less – per 100 grams of the product. That's equivalent to four per cent fat. Beware of products labelled 'lite' or 'reduced fat'. Many low-fat spreads and dressings still contain large amounts of fat, so make sure you always check the nutrition panel carefully.

While the four per cent rule is a good yardstick,

there are exceptions. If you remove the skin and visible fat, then lean beef, lamb, pork, venison, poultry and fish are totally acceptable. The other exceptions are products such as mustard, curry powder and so on where you will only be eating minimal amounts. Use your discretion.

# Don't eat these foods if you want to lose weight

Unless included in the diet menus or recipes, the following foods are strictly forbidden while following the diet, though some exceptions are made for vegetarians.

Butter, margarine, Flora, low-fat spreads containing more than four per cent fat, or any similar products.

Cream, soured cream, Gold top, whole milk etc.

Lard, oil (all types), dripping, suet, etc.

Fried foods of any kind (except dry-fried).

Fat or skin from all meats, poultry etc.

All cheese (except low-fat cottage cheese).

All nuts (except chestnuts).

Goose and all fatty meats.

Meat products, e.g. Scotch eggs, pork pie, faggots, black pudding, haggis, liver sausage, pâté.

All types of sausages and salami.

Sauces and dressings containing cream, whole milk or eggs.

Cakes, sweet biscuits, pastries (including savoury
   pastries), sponge puddings etc.
Chocolate, toffees, fudge, caramel, butterscotch.
Savoury biscuits and crackers.
Lemon curd, peanut butter and chocolate spread.
Marzipan.
Cocoa and cocoa products, Horlicks and chocolate
   drinks.
Crisps and snacks.
Avocado pears and olives.
Egg products, e.g. quiches, egg custard, crème brûlée,
   crème caramel.
Ice cream made with real cream.

NB Low-fat branded products that contain a
maximum of four per cent are permitted. However,
just because something is low in fat, it does not mean
that you can eat it in unlimited quantities. If you
want to lose weight, it is important to follow the diet
as stated.


# Avoiding the Pitfalls

Inevitably on any weight-loss regime there are people
who fall by the wayside or who find it hard to lose
weight. There are a number of reasons for this, but
if you follow the advice in this book, then this should
not apply to you. Make sure that you don't fall into
into any of the following traps.

## The Top Ten Reasons Why People Don't Lose Weight

1 *They eat too much*. In recent clinical studies, slim and overweight people were asked to make a written record of their daily intake of food and drink. While the slim people accurately recorded their consumption, the overweight ones underestimated how much they ate by 33 per cent!

2 *They* do *too little*. Overweight people tend to be less active than slim people. This is mostly due to the extra effort required to be active because they are carrying 'excess baggage'. The good news is that because of that extra weight, they do not need to do as much exercise as a slimmer person to achieve the same energy expenditure. The key is to do as much as you can, as often as you can.

3 *They don't understand the diet rules*. Dieters often remember only the parts of the diet that they like and amalgamate them to form their own special version! Each diet has its own individual formula, so re-read the instructions and re-read the list of forbidden foods on pages 47–48 – and stick to the rules.

4 *They break the rules*. Through lack of willpower, dieters sometimes simply break the rules and cheat! Eating between meals is forbidden in the diet in this book. The only exception is you can save your dessert from your evening meal to have as a snack earlier or later in the evening.

5  *They exercise on an empty stomach.* Obviously, we should not exercise on a full stomach, but it is important to put some 'fuel' back into our 'energy tank', say, half an hour before an aerobic workout. This will encourage maximum fat-burning to take place. If you exercise first thing in the morning, drink your 150ml (¼ pint) glass of orange juice 15 minutes before you start. If you plan to go to an exercise class straight from your place of work, have your fruit dessert from your evening meal half an hour *before* the class. But, remember, you can't have another dessert later!

6  *They are not highly motivated.* Unless you have a reason for wanting to lose weight you are unlikely to succeed. Read Chapter 4 carefully for tips to get yourself into the right frame of mind.

7  *They don't understand what made them over-weight in the first place.* We gain weight because we take in more calories than the body needs. That is an undisputed fact. Unless we accept this and adjust our food intake and our energy output accordingly, we will not lose weight. *We* make ourselves over-weight – nobody else does.

8  *They don't eat enough.* The body requires a certain number of calories to enable it to function efficiently. If we give it too little food, the body switches to 'emergency mode' so that it can survive on very few calories. This has the effect of drastically slowing down our rate of weight loss. So, if you are eating only one small meal a day and wondering why

you are not losing weight, that's the reason why. Start eating three meals a day, and you'll be amazed at how much weight you start to lose.

9  *They eat as much low-fat or fat-free food as they like and think they won't gain weight.* A great deal of confusion arises here. People sometimes over-simplify the diet and think that they can eat as much food as they like as long as it's low in fat. If only it were that simple! The truth is that all foods contain calories, and if we eat too many calories we will gain weight. However, some foods are utilised by the body more efficiently than others. High-fat foods are badly utilised, resulting in a more speedy weight gain – that's why we keep their consumption to a minimum. But let there be no misunderstanding. Even if a food contains no fat – like boiled sweets for instance – we can certainly gain weight if we eat them in addition to our daily calorie allowance or, in this case, the diet as detailed in this book.

10  *They eat up the leftovers.* A dieter may be sticking to the diet like a saint, but then when the children leave food on their plates, the old maxim, 'let's not waste anything – think of the starving millions', takes over. Often we eat leftovers without actually realising we're eating them! Train your children to discard their leftovers *before* you get to clear away their plates!

# Getting started on the Plan

Choose a day when you will start the Plan and clear out all the high-fat foods from your kitchen. You are going to get rid of your old bad habits and replace them with new, healthy ones. Remember, to maximise your fat loss you need to combine low-fat eating with exercise. Here's what you do.

## The Diet

Follow the diet instructions, selecting three meals a day from the menus listed for breakfast, lunch and dinner. Dinner is three courses, so you can have a starter, a main course and a dessert. You can save your dessert to have as a snack later in the evening, or earlier if you wish.

## The Exercises

To achieve maximum fat-burning you need to do some aerobic exercise for 10–20 minutes on five days each week. Aerobic exercise is any form of exercise that makes you slightly out of breath such as brisk walking or jogging. If you prefer, you can attend an aerobics class or work out at home to an aerobics video. See Chapter 8 for more information.

In addition, ideally try to practise the toning workout in Chapter 8 every day if possible. The workout contains three individual routines, so start with the Elementary routine and progress according to your ability. Each routine takes only ten minutes and, practised regularly, will dramatically strengthen your abdominal and postural muscles.

## Ten Tips to Make This Plan Work for You

1  Follow the diet instructions and select from the menu suggestions. You *will* lose weight if you stick to these rules.

2  Eat three meals a day and don't skip breakfast.

3  Do eat sufficient at mealtimes to satisfy your appetite. Fill up on low-calorie salads and vegetables if you still feel hungry. This way, you won't be tempted to snack later.

4  You don't have to eat a starter with your evening meal if you don't want it. It's there to help fill you up quicker so that you are not tempted to overeat with the main course. A long, low-calorie drink will do the same job, so take one before every meal.

5  Do not eat between meals, although you are allowed to save your dessert to eat as a supper later in the evening, or earlier if you wish.

6  If you do feel desperately hungry between meals, eat carrot or celery sticks, but do try to break the habit of snacking between meals.

7  If you have a bad day and stray from the diet, don't throw in the towel and waste all the effort you have put in so far. Instead, go back to the diet and eat the next meal (even if you're not hungry) and get back on track. Skipping meals will only lead to bingeing, and that's just what we want to avoid.

8   Any form of exercise burns calories and helps maintain your muscle mass. Remember, muscle needs calories to sustain it. Regular aerobic exercise will help you to lose weight faster and more efficiently. So, in addition to the exercises in Chapter 8, do try working out at home to a video or go to your local Diet and Fitness class (see back of book for details).

9   Try to be more physically active in your everyday life. Look for ways you can be more energetic and get into a new, more active lifestyle.

10   Ask a partner or friend to take a photograph of you before you start. There's no need to show it to anyone else. Just keep it safe so that you can get it out later and check your progress. Also, take time to measure yourself with a tape measure each week and keep a record. I promise, when you see those inches disappearing, you'll be glad you did.

# 6

# The Complete Flat Stomach Plan Diet

This Complete Flat Stomach Plan Diet offers a wide variety of menu suggestions that all the family can enjoy. You will find lots of quick and easy options, including ready-made meals, as well as recipes for the more adventurous cook. Read the instructions below before you start. Stick to the rules, don't skip meals, and be aware of the benefits you will be achieving for both your figure and your health.

## Diet Instructions

Eat three meals a day, selecting from the breakfast, lunch and dinner menus listed. Do not eat between meals, but if you feel really peckish, fill up on sticks of carrots, celery, cucumber and peppers.

Men over 5ft 8in (1.78m) or who are involved in heavy physical labour may increase the quantities by 25 per cent.

## Daily Nutritional Requirements

In selecting your menus, each day try to incorporate the following *minimum* quantities:

175g (6oz) protein food (fish, poultry, meat, cottage cheese).

350g (12oz) vegetables (including salad).

350g (12oz) fresh fruit (including fruit juice).

175g (6oz) carbohydrate (bread, cereals, potatoes, rice, pasta).

## Diet Notes

**Bread** should be wholemeal whenever possible. For guidance, one slice of regular bread from a large thin-sliced loaf weighs 25g (1oz). A slice from a large medium-sliced loaf weighs 40g (1½oz). Unless otherwise specified in the menus, one slice equals 25g (1oz). Light bread means low-calorie brands such as Nimble.

**Cottage cheese** should be the low-fat variety. Flavoured varieties are acceptable, but check the nutritional panel for fat content and avoid ones with added cream.

**Diet yogurt** means low-fat, low-calorie brands. 1 × 150g (5oz) pot should contain no more than 70 calories.

**Gravy** may be taken with dinner menus provided it is made with gravy powder or low-fat granules. Do not add meat juices from the roasting tin unless you first discard the fat.

**1 piece fresh fruit** means 1 average apple or 1 orange

etc., or approximately 115g (4oz) any fruit such as grapes, pineapple, strawberries etc. Do not eat fruit between meals.

**Pasta and rice** are restricted to 50g (2oz) uncooked weight per portion unless otherwise specified. Choose wholemeal varieties where possible.

**Unlimited vegetables** includes potatoes as well as all other vegetables provided they are cooked and served without fat.

## Sauces and Dressings

The following may be consumed freely:

Brown sauce
Chilli sauce
Fat-free salad dressings
Horseradish sauce
Lemon juice
Marmite
Mint sauce
Mustard
Oil-free vinaigrette
Soy sauce
Tomato ketchup
Vinegar (any type)
Worcester sauce

For other sauces and dressings, check the nutrition panel on the label before you buy and select those with 4g or less fat per 100g of product. Exceptions are foods of which you will use only tiny amounts.

## Daily Allowance

- 450ml (³⁄₄ pint) skimmed or semi-skimmed milk.
- 150ml (¹⁄₄ pint) unsweetened orange, grapefruit or apple juice.
- One unit alcoholic drink for women, two units for men.
- Tea and coffee may be drunk freely, using milk from allowance. Diet drinks and water are also unlimited.
- Unlimited salad and vegetables, cooked and served without fat, may be eaten with lunch and dinner.

# The Diet

Here is a list of the various menu sections under which you'll find a selection of meal options. Choose one breakfast, one lunch and one dinner menu each day.

### Breakfasts

Cereal Breakfasts
Fruit Breakfasts
Cooked and Continental Breakfasts

### Lunches

Salads
Salad Specials
Home-made Sandwiches
Pitta Bread Pockets

Hot Sandwiches
Prepacked Sandwiches
Quick and Easy Snack Lunches
Jacket Potato Lunches
Gourmet Lunches

## Dinners

### *Starters*
Quick and Easy Starters
Instant Soup Starters: Vegetarian
Instant Soup Starters: Non Vegetarian
Gourmet Starters

### *Main Courses*
Basic Main Courses
Ready-made Meals for One
Ready-made Meals for Two
Ready-made and Quick and Easy Meals for
Vegetarians
Quick and Easy Cook-in-Sauce Meals
Simple Meat Recipes
Simple Poultry Recipes
Simple Fish Recipes
Simple Vegetarian Recipes
Gourmet Recipes
Vegetable Accompaniments

### *Desserts*
Quick and Easy Desserts
Instant Desserts
Gourmet Desserts
Cakes and Loaves

# Breakfasts

*Select any one*

## Cereal Breakfasts

Served with milk from allowance where appropriate

- 25g (1oz) any cereal with 1 teaspoon sugar, plus 1 slice wholemeal toast spread with 2 teaspoons marmalade or honey.
- 25g (1oz) muesli with 1 teaspoon sugar, plus 225g (8oz) strawberries or 1 sliced banana.
- 25g (1oz) muesli mixed with 1 × 200g (7oz) Muller-light yogurt.
- 40g (1½oz) Grape Nuts with 1 teaspoon sugar, plus 1 sliced banana.
- 50g (2oz) Kellogg's All-Bran with 1 teaspoon sugar, plus 115g (4oz) strawberries or 1 chopped apple.
- 40g (1½oz) Weight Watchers Perfect Balance with 1 teaspoon sugar, plus 1 sliced banana.
- 50g (2oz) Kellogg's Bran Buds with 1 teaspoon sugar, plus 115g (4oz) any fresh fruit.
- 2 Nestlé Shredded Wheat with 2 teaspoons sugar, plus 115g (4oz) any fresh fruit.
- 40g (1½oz) sultana bran, plus either 1 sliced banana or 1 × 150g (5oz) pot low-fat natural yogurt.
- 50g (2oz) Kellogg's Special K with 1 teaspoon sugar, plus 50g (2oz) seedless grapes.
- 50g (2oz) cornflakes with 1 teaspoon sugar, plus 115g (4oz) any fresh fruit.

- 50g (2oz) fruit and fibre cereal with 1 teaspoon sugar.
- 2 Weetabix with 1 teaspoon sugar, plus 1 sliced banana
- 65g (2½oz) Kellogg's Frosties.
- 65g (2½oz) Kellogg's Rice Krispies with 1 teaspoon sugar.
- Austrian Muesli (see recipe, page 97).
- Porridge (see recipe, pages 97–8).

## Fruit Breakfasts

- 4 pieces any fresh fruit.
- 1 banana plus 1 × 200g (7oz) Mullerlight yogurt.
- 5 canned prunes in natural juice plus 1 × 150g (5oz) low-fat natural yogurt.
- 1 whole fresh grapefruit, plus 2 × 150g (5oz) diet yogurts.
- 1 wedge melon topped with 115g (4oz) grapes and served with 1 × 150g (5oz) diet yogurt.
- 200g (7oz) any stewed fruit cooked without sugar and topped with 1 × 150g (5oz) diet yogurt.
- 4 apricots soaked overnight in herbal or regular tea and served with 1 × 150g (5oz) diet yogurt or low-fat fromage frais.
- 300g (11oz) canned grapefruit segments in natural juice.
- 1 × 200g (7oz) can green figs in syrup, topped with 1 × 150g (5oz) diet yogurt.
- 1 × 200g (7oz) can Tesco Breakfast Apricots in Apple Juice, topped with 1 × 150g (5oz) diet yogurt.

- 1 × 300g (11oz) can Tesco Breakfast Compote in Apple Juice, topped with 1 × 150g (5oz) diet yogurt.
- 1 × 220g (7½oz) can Del Monte Sliced Pineapple in Natural Juice, topped with 75g (3oz) low-fat fromage frais.
- 1 × 213g (7¼oz) can Sainsbury's Fruit Cocktail in Grape Juice, topped with 1 × 150g (5oz) diet yogurt.
- 1 × 205g (7oz) can Sainsbury's Apricot Halves in Apple and Apricot Juice, topped with 1 × 150g (5oz) low-fat fromage frais.
- 1 × 298g (11oz) can Sainsbury's Spanish Mandarin Orange Segments in Natural Juice, topped with 1 × 150g (5oz) orange-flavoured diet yogurt.
- 1 × 250g (9oz) can Marks and Spencer Sliced Mango in Syrup, plus 1 Marks and Spencer Lite Fromage Frais.
- 1 × 300g (11oz) can Marks and Spencer Exotic Fruit Salad in light Syrup, plus 1 Marks and Spencer Lite Fromage Frais.

## Cooked and Continental Breakfasts

- ½ fresh grapefruit, plus 1 slice wholemeal toast topped with 3 turkey rashers (e.g. Mattessons), grilled, and 2 sliced tomatoes.
- ½ fresh grapefruit, plus 1 small poached or boiled egg served with 1 slice wholemeal toast spread with Marmite.
- 2 slices wholemeal toast spread with 3 teaspoons marmalade or honey.

- 1 slice wholemeal toast spread with 2 teaspoons marmalade or honey, plus 2 pieces fresh fruit of your choice.
- Contents of 1 × 200g (7oz) can tomatoes well boiled and reduced to a creamy consistency served on 1 slice wholemeal toast and topped with 2 grilled turkey rashers.
- Contents of 1 × 200g (7oz) can baked beans served on 1 slice wholemeal toast, plus 1 × 150g (5oz) diet yogurt.
- 1 × 50g (2oz) wholemeal roll spread with HP or Branston Fruity Sauce and filled with 1 well-grilled turkey rasher and a sliced tomato.
- 1 × 50g (2oz) wholemeal roll spread with horse-radish sauce and filled with 25g (1oz) wafer thin pastrami.
- 40g (1½oz) wholemeal toast spread with HP or Branston Fruity Sauce and topped with 25g (1oz) wafer thin ham and 25g (1oz) wafer thin pastrami.
- 2 grilled turkey rashers served with 115g (4oz) baked beans and 2 grilled tomatoes, plus 1 piece fresh fruit or 1 × 150g (5oz) diet yogurt.
- 1 wholemeal muffin plus 1 piece fresh fruit.
- 1 bagel toasted and served with 2 teaspoons jam or marmalade.
- 1 whole grapefruit, plus 2 grilled turkey rashers, served with 1 egg dry-fried in a non-stick pan, 1 slice toasted light bread and 1 grilled tomato.
- 2 grilled turkey rashers and unlimited grilled tomatoes and mushrooms cooked without fat, plus 1 slice wholemeal toast.

# Lunches

*Select any one*

## Salad Lunches

Be adventurous with your salads. Use any of the following ingredients in unlimited quantities if eaten at one sitting. Make your own dressings by choosing from the recipes on pages 242–4, or choose branded low-fat, oil-free or fat-free dressings. Just look at the labels and select those with four per cent or less fat. Allow 2 tablespoons of dressing per person.

Asparagus
Beansprouts
Beetroot, grated raw or cooked and sliced
Carrots, grated raw
Cucumber
Courgettes
Lettuce, all varieties
Mushrooms, all varieties
Mustard cress
Onions, all varieties
Peas, all varieties
Peppers, green, red or yellow
Sweetcorn
Tomatoes
Watercress

Make a large salad using any combination of the above items and serve with:

75g (3oz) boiled new potatoes
OR
1 slice wholemeal bread
OR
1 × 30g (1½oz) packet The Low Fat Snack Co. 99%
Fat Free Potato Crisp Waffles
PLUS
*one* of the items listed below and 1 piece fresh fruit
or 1 × 150g (5oz) diet yogurt.

**Select any *one* or combine two half-portions**

- 115g (4oz) low-fat cottage cheese.
- 75g (3oz) prawns, shelled and cooked.
- 75g (3oz) canned tuna (in brine) or salmon or mackerel or sardines (in tomato sauce).
- 175g (6oz) chicken leg (weighed with bone), no skin.
- 75g (3oz) wafer thin chicken or turkey (any brand).
- 75g (3oz) Asda, Safeway, Sainsbury's or Tesco Wafer Thin Pastrami.
- 75g (3oz) Bernard Matthews Wafer Thin Turkey Tikka Masala.
- 75g (3oz) Bernard Matthews Turkey Breast Roll.
- 75g (3oz) Asda Wafer Thin Smoked Ham.
- 75g (3oz) Marks and Spencer Wafer Thin Honey Roast Ham.
- 75g (3oz) Marks and Spencer Oak Smoked Danish Ham.
- 75g (3oz) Marks and Spencer Wafer Thin Chargrilled Ham.

## Salad Specials

- Rice salad: 25g (1oz) (uncooked weight) brown rice cooked and mixed with 25g (1oz) chickpeas, 25g (1oz) red kidney beans, unlimited peas, sweetcorn, chopped peppers, chopped tomatoes, diced cucumber and oil-free dressing of your choice.
- Bean Salad (see recipe, page 98).
- Cheese, Prawn and Asparagus Salad (see recipe, page 99).
- Fruit and Chicken Salad (see recipe, pages 99–100).
- Prawn and Pasta Salad (see recipe, page 100).
- Red Kidney Bean Salad (see recipe, page 101).

## Sandwich Lunches

### Home-made Sandwiches

Use 2 slices from a large wholemeal loaf OR 4 slices of light bread OR 6 Ryvitas. Spread with mustard, horseradish sauce, pickle or any low-fat sauce or dressing that is less than 4 per cent fat (butter, margarine and low-fat spreads are strictly forbidden). Fill with unlimited chopped salad and *one* of the items below.

NB Wafer thin meats are a real boon for the slimmer as even a small serving looks quite generous. While this type is recommended, any sliced lean meat is fine – but watch the quantity, as you don't feel you are eating as much!

- 50g (2oz) wafer thin ham, chicken, turkey or pastrami.
- 75g (3oz) low-fat cottage cheese (any flavour).
- 25g (1oz) low-fat cottage cheese and 1 sliced banana.
- 50g (2oz) canned tuna (in brine), salmon or sardines (in tomato sauce).
- 50g (2oz) prawns or mackerel.
- 1 hard-boiled egg, chopped and mixed with 1 tablespoon low-fat natural yogurt and 1 tablespoon branded reduced-oil salad dressing.

## Pitta Bread Pockets

Split one pitta bread and spread with very low-fat dressing. Fill with chopped salad and *one* of the following:

- 50g (2oz) wafer thin cooked ham, chicken, turkey or pastrami.
- 50g (2oz) cooked chicken, chopped and mixed with 1 tablespoon low-fat natural yogurt, 1 tablespoon reduced-oil salad dressing (any brand) plus ½ teaspoon curry powder.
- 50g (2oz) chicken tikka (ready-prepared or home-made).
- 75g (3oz) low-fat cottage cheese mixed with chopped salad vegetables.
- 50g (2oz) low-fat cottage cheese (any flavour) mixed with 50g (2oz) low-fat coleslaw.
- 50g (2oz) canned tuna (in brine) mixed with 1 tablespoon reduced-oil salad dressing (any brand) and 50g (2oz) sweetcorn.

## Hot Sandwiches

- Spread 2 medium slices wholemeal toast with Branston or HP Fruity Sauce. Fill with 2 slices Danepak Lean and Low Rindless Prime Back Bacon, well grilled.
- Halve a 50g (2oz) piece of French stick and spread each half with tomato ketchup. Fill with 25g (1oz) cooked ham and 50g (2oz) pineapple or 25g (1oz) mackerel in tomato sauce. Bake in a pre-heated oven at 180°C, 350°F or Gas mark 4 for 4–5 minutes. Serve with salad.
- Micro Sandwich (see recipe, pages 101–2).
- Club Sandwich (see recipe, pages 102–3).

## Prepacked Sandwiches

For those who go out to work, ready-made, pre-packed sandwiches can be a tremendous help and there is now a wide variety to choose from. Below is a selection of low-fat sandwiches from three retail companies. Some contain slightly more than 4 per cent fat (maximum 4.5 per cent) but this extra amount of fat is so tiny that it will not adversely affect your progress on the diet.

With some sandwiches I have allowed additional fruit and/or a diet yogurt to make up the number of calories you are allowed for lunch. If no fruit or yogurt is included, this means the sandwich already contains sufficient calories.

## Asda

- 1 pack Light Tuna and Cucumber sandwiches, plus 1 piece fresh fruit and 1 × 150g (5oz) diet yogurt.
- 1 pack Light Smoked Ham Salad sandwiches, plus 1 piece fresh fruit or 1 × 150g (5oz) diet yogurt.

## Boots Shapers

- 1 pack Egg Salad sandwiches, plus 1 piece fresh fruit and 1 × 150g (5oz) diet yogurt.
- 1 pack Greek Style Salad with Feta Cheese and Yogurt Dressing sandwiches, plus 1 piece fresh fruit and 1 × 150g (5oz) diet yogurt.
- 1 pack Prawn, Apple and Celery with Soft Cheese sandwiches, plus 1 piece fresh fruit and 1 × 150g (5oz) diet yogurt.
- 1 pack Bacon, Lettuce and Tomato sandwiches, plus 1 piece fresh fruit and 1 × 150g (5oz) diet yogurt.
- 1 pack Smoked Ham and Cottage Cheese with Lettuce, Chives and Mayonnaise sandwiches, plus 1 piece fresh fruit and 1 × 150g (5oz) diet yogurt.
- 1 mixed pack Smoked Ham/Soft Cheese and Pineapple with Lettuce sandwiches, plus 1 piece fresh fruit and 1 × 150g (5oz) diet yogurt.
- 1 pack Italian Style Chicken and Fresh Basil with Little Gem sandwiches, plus 1 piece fresh fruit and 1 × 150g (5oz) diet yogurt.
- 1 pack Smoked Ham Salad with Mustard Dressing sandwiches, plus 1 piece fresh fruit and 1 × 150g (5oz) diet yogurt.
- 1 pack Roast Chicken and Back Bacon with

Tomato and Lettuce sandwiches, plus 1 piece fresh fruit and 1 × 150g (5oz) diet yogurt.

- 1 pack Turkey, Ham and Coleslaw sandwiches, plus 1 piece fresh fruit and 1 × 150g (5oz) diet yogurt.
- 1 pack Turkey and Chinese Leaf with Sage and Onion Mayonnaise sandwiches, plus 1 piece fresh fruit and 1 × 150g (5oz) diet yogurt.
- 1 pack Salmon with Cucumber, Lettuce and Mayonnaise sandwiches, plus 1 piece fresh fruit and 1 × 150g (5oz) diet yogurt.
- 1 mixed pack Chicken and Ham/Chicken and Coleslaw/Chicken and Sweetcorn sandwiches.
- 1 pack Two Mini New York Style Bagels: Barbecued Chicken with Barbecue Relish and Tomato/ Chargrill Flavoured Chicken and Peppers with Garlic Dressing.
- 1 Ham Salad Bap, plus 1 piece fresh fruit and 1 × 150g (5oz) diet yogurt.

### Marks and Spencer

- 1 pack Wafer Thin Smoked Turkey and Coleslaw sandwiches, plus 1 piece fresh fruit or 1 × 150g (5oz) diet yogurt.
- 1 pack Chicken and Lemon Mayonnaise sandwiches, plus 1 piece fresh fruit or 1 × 150g (5oz) diet yogurt.
- 1 pack Lean Danish Ham and Salad sandwiches, plus 1 piece fresh fruit or 1 × 150g (5oz) diet yogurt.
- 1 pack Egg and Salad sandwiches, plus 1 piece fresh fruit or 1 × 150g (5oz) diet yogurt.

## Quick and Easy Snack Lunches

- 1 × 200g (7oz) pot Mullerice Dairy Rice with Apples in Syrup, plus 1 apple.
- 3 pieces fresh fruit (350g/12oz total) plus 1 × 150g (5oz) Safeway Toffee Flavoured Low Fat Yogurt.
- 1 sachet Batchelors Slim a Soup plus 1 × 200g (7oz) pot Mullerice Dairy Rice with Caramel and 1 piece fresh fruit.
- 1 sachet Batchelors Slim a Soup plus 2 pieces fresh fruit and 1 Safeway Crème Caramel.
- 1 sachet Batchelors Slim a Soup or Weight Watchers Instant Soup, plus 2 pieces fresh fruit and 2 × 150g (2 × 5oz) diet yogurts.
- 1 sachet Batchelors Slim a Soup, plus 2 slices wholemeal bread spread with reduced-oil salad dressing and filled with salad and 50g (2oz) low-fat cottage cheese.
- 1 × 405g (14oz) can Heinz Country Vegetable Soup.
- 1 × 405g (14oz) can Heinz Winter Vegetable Wholesoup.
- 1 Golden Wonder Pot Light Chinese Chicken, plus 2 pieces fresh fruit.
- 1 Golden Wonder Pot Light Chicken and Mushroom, plus 2 × 150g (5oz) diet yogurts.
- 1 Golden Wonder Pot Light Italien Chicken, plus 1 piece fresh fruit and 1 × 150g (5oz) diet yogurt.
- 1 × 295g (11oz) can Heinz Weight Watchers Wholesome Soup, plus 40g (1½oz) wholemeal bread and 1 piece fresh fruit.
- 1 × 295g (11oz) can Heinz Weight Watchers Lentil

and Carrot Soup, plus 40g (1½oz) wholemeal bread and 1 piece fresh fruit.

- ½ × 295g (11oz) can Campbell's Condensed Half Fat Tomato Soup, plus 40g (1½oz) wholemeal bread.
- ½ × 295g (11oz) can Campbell's Condensed Half Fat Mushroom Soup, plus 1 × 150g (5oz) diet yogurt.
- 1 × 425g (15oz) can Baxters Healthy Choice Chicken and Vegetable Soup, plus 40g (1½oz) wholemeal bread.
- ½ × 425g (15oz) can Baxters Carrot and Butter Bean Soup, plus 40g (1½oz) wholemeal bread and 1 piece fresh fruit.
- ½ × 425g (15oz) can Baxters Country Garden Soup, plus 40g (1½oz) wholemeal bread and 1 piece fresh fruit.
- Marks and Spencer Lite Chicken Salad with Coleslaw, plus 1 Marks and Spencer Very Low Fat Lite Yogurt.
- Marks and Spencer Pasta Salad with Sweetcorn, plus 1 × 150g (5oz) diet yogurt.
- Marks and Spencer Deep Filled Jacket Potato with Fresh Vegetables and Chilli Sauce, plus 1 Marks and Spencer Fruit Cocktail.

## Jacket Potato Lunches

1 × 225g (8oz) jacket potato with *one* of the following
toppings, served with salad.

- 75g (3oz) low-fat coleslaw mixed with 10 sultanas
  and 1 × 150g (5oz) diet yogurt.
- 75g (3oz) canned tuna in brine, drained and mixed
  with 1 teaspoon reduced-oil salad dressing.
- 50g (2oz) prawns mixed with 50g (2oz) sweetcorn,
  1 tablespoon reduced-oil salad dressing and 1
  tablespoon tomato ketchup.
- 50g (2oz) cooked chicken, cut into cubes and
  mixed with 75g (3oz) low-fat natural yogurt and 1
  teaspoon curry powder.
- 50g (2oz) cooked chicken mixed with 1 tablespoon
  low-fat natural yogurt, 1 tablespoon reduced-oil
  salad dressing and red and green peppers.
- 50g (2oz) turkey rashers, chopped and dry-fried
  with 1 small chopped onion and 4 mushrooms.
  Add 2 tablespoons chilli sauce and mix well.
- 115g (4oz) baked beans mixed with ¼ teaspoon
  chilli powder.
- 200g (7oz) spaghetti hoops, plus 2 tomatoes.
- 115g (4oz) low-fat cottage cheese with pineapple
  or chives.
- 115g (4oz) low-fat cottage cheese mixed with red
  and green peppers.
- 50g (2oz) low-fat cottage cheese mixed with 25g
  (1oz) tuna in brine and 1 tablespoon low-fat salad
  dressing.
- 50g (2oz) low-fat cottage cheese mixed with 25g

(1oz) canned red kidney beans and 25g (1oz) canned sweetcorn.

- 38g (1½oz) Shape 97% Fat Free Smoked Ham Spread or Fat Free Spread with Cheese, plus 1 piece fresh fruit.
- 75g (3oz) The 'Fresh Dip' Company Onion and Garlic Dip or Cucumber and Mint Dip.
- 115g (4oz) Shape Virtually Fat Free Cottage Cheese (any flavour).
- 1 × 170g (6oz) jar Heinz Weight Watchers Potato Toppers Sweet and Sour Chicken.
- 1 × 170g (6oz) jar Heinz Weight Watchers Potato Toppers Chicken and Vegetable Masala.
- Creamy Topping for Baked Potatoes (see recipe, page 103).

## Gourmet Lunches

- Potato and Leek Soup (see recipe, pages 103–4) plus 1 slice bread or toast and 1 piece fresh fruit.
- Winter Warmer Soup (see recipe, pages 104–5) plus 25g (1oz) crusty bread.
- Chicken Drumstick Surprise (see recipe, page 105) served with unlimited salad and 1 piece fresh fruit.
- Baked Potatoes with Apple (see recipe, page 106).
- Smoked Haddock and Potato Boats (see recipe, page 107).

# Dinners

*Select one starter, one main course and one dessert*

In this selection of dinner options I've tried to cater for everyone – from the gourmet cook to the too-busy-to-cook person who wants to eat something hot that's quick to prepare. By popular request I have also included some ready-made meals.

Feel free to add extra vegetables or salad ingredients to your main course to help fill you up. It is important that you leave the table feeling more than satisfied. If you do, then you'll be less likely to cheat later.

# Starters

*Select any one*

## Quick and Easy Starters

- Wedge of melon sprinkled with ground ginger.
- Half a grapefruit.
- Half a galia melon or one quarter honeydew melon topped with 40g (1½oz) prawns in a fat-free dressing.
- Half a melon topped with 50g (2oz) strawberries.
- Crudités (sticks or sprigs of cucumber, carrots, cauliflower and peppers) served with Garlic and Mint Yogurt Dip (see recipe, page 244).

- Marks and Spencer Stuffed Vine Leaves (2 per serving).

## Instant Soup Starters: Vegetarian

*Heinz*

- 1 × 200g (7oz) serving Potato and Leek Soup.
- 1 × 200g (7oz) serving Winter Vegetable Wholesoup.
- 1 × 200g (7oz) serving Country Vegetable Wholesoup.

*John Lusty*
- 1 × 200g (7oz) serving French Onion Soup.

*Marks and Spencer*
- ½ can Minestrone Soup.

*New Covent Garden Soup Company*
- 1 × 200g (7oz) serving Fresh Lentil Soup with Winter Vegetables.
- 1 × 200g (7oz) serving Fresh Minestrone Soup.

## Instant soup starters: non-vegetarian

*Becas*

- 1 × 200g (7oz) serving Duck and Cranberry Soup.

*Campbell's*
- ½ × 295g (11oz) can Condensed Half Fat Chicken Soup.

*Heinz*
- 1 × 150g (5oz) serving Oxtail Soup.
- 1 × 150g (5oz) serving Scotch Broth Traditional Farmhouse Soup.

*John Lusty*
- 1 × 200g (7oz) serving Crab Bisque.
- 1 × 200g (7oz) serving Chicken Consommé.

## Gourmet Starters

- Cucumber Boats with Tuna (page 108).
- Garlic Mushrooms (page 109).
- Low-fat Hummus with Crudités (page 110).
- Melon Salad (page 111).
- Prawn or Crab Cocktail (page 112).
- Smoked Mackerel Pâté (page 112).
- Cream of Courgette Soup (page 113).
- Fresh Vegetable Soup (page 114).
- Gazpacho (page 114).
- Low-fat Creamy Potato and Parsley Soup (page 115).
- Pea and Lettuce Soup (page 116).

# Main Courses

*Select any one*

## Basic Main Courses

- 115g (4oz) roast lamb or beef served with Dry-roast Potatoes and Dry-roast Parsnips (see recipes, pages 210–11), with extra vegetables and fat-free gravy, mint or horseradish sauce.
- 3 lamb chops (225g/8oz cooked weight including bone), grilled with all fat removed and served with mint sauce, 115g (4oz) potatoes creamed with low-fat natural yogurt, plus unlimited vegetables and fat-free gravy.
- 175g (6oz) pork chop (cooked weight including bone), grilled with all fat removed, served with 50g (2oz) apple sauce, 50g (2oz) sage and onion stuffing, unlimited new potatoes and vegetables plus fat-free gravy.
- 175g (6oz) calf's or lamb's liver, braised with onions in a fat-free gravy, served with 115g (4oz) potatoes creamed with low-fat natural yogurt, plus unlimited vegetables.
- 175g (6oz) roast chicken served with Dry-roast Potatoes (see recipe, pages 210–11), plus unlimited vegetables and fat-free gravy.
- 150g (5oz) roast pork served with Dry-roast Potatoes (see recipe, pages 210–11) plus unlimited vegetables, fat-free gravy and 50g (2oz) apple sauce.
- 175g (6oz) chopped chicken, stir-fried in soy sauce

with onions, mushrooms and black pepper and
served on a bed of boiled rice (50g/2oz uncooked
weight per person).

- 115g (4oz) fillet steak topped with green peppercorns in low-fat fromage frais and served with 175g
(6oz) jacket potato topped with low-fat fromage
frais sprinkled with chives, plus unlimited peas,
tomatoes and mushrooms.
- 225g (8oz) any white fish steamed, grilled or micro-
waved, served with 115g (4oz) potatoes mashed
with low-fat natural yogurt (no butter) plus unlimited vegetables and tomato ketchup.

## Ready-made Meals For One

Prepacked meals are useful for those people who
don't want the hassle of cooking. Nowadays, there
is a vast choice available and most of them are
microwaveable. However, if you eat these often, it
can get expensive and if, like me, you have a large
appetite, then you're probably still going to feel
hungry afterwards. The answer is to cook lots of
healthy vegetables to accompany the meal. These
will help fill you up so you won't be tempted to
nibble later and will also provide you with extra
nutrients. Don't forget to have a starter and a
dessert.

### Asda
- Pasta Bolognese (300g/11oz pack).
- Spaghetti Bolognese (300g/11oz pack).

## *Findus Lean Cuisine*

- Chicken and Broccoli Pasta (230g/8½oz pack).
- Chicken à l'Orange (252g/9oz pack).
- Chicken and Ham Lasagne Verdi (275g/10oz pack).
- Chicken and Prawn Creole (230g/8½oz pack).
- Glazed Chicken with Rice (272g/10oz pack).
- Kashmiri Chicken Curry (262g/9½oz pack).
- Lean Beef Lasagne (300g/11oz pack).
- Mediterranean Tuna Pasta (230g/ 8½oz pack).
- Prawn Curry (291g/11oz pack).
- Smoked Ham and Mushroom Tagliatelle (230g/ 8½oz pack).
- Spanish Paella (265g/9½oz pack).

## *Heinz Weight Watchers*

- Beef Lasagne (295g/11oz pack).
- Menu Plus Chicken Supreme (300g/11oz pack).
- Pasta Plus Chicken and Broccoli Pasta Bake (305g/11oz pack).
- Seafood Plus Salmon Mornay with Broccoli (290g/ 10½oz pack).
- Tagliatelle Carbonara.

## *Marks and Spencer*

- Chicken Chow Mein (200g/7oz pack).
- Kedgeree (200g/7oz pack).
- Chilli Con Carne with Rice.
- Chicken Casserole.
- Cod in Parsley Sauce.

● Chargrilled Tomato, Cod and Pasta.

### Safeway
● Chicken and Cashew Nuts (300g/11oz pack).
● Chilli con Carne with Rice (300g/11oz pack).
● Chinese Style Chicken with Egg Fried Rice (225g/ 8oz pack).
● Spaghetti Bolognese (300g/11oz pack).
● Sweet and Sour Pork with Rice (250g/9oz pack).

### Sainsbury's
● Long Life Lancashire Hot Pot (300g/11oz pack).

## Ready-made Meals for Two

● Asda Chilli Con Carne (454g/16oz pack).
● Marks and Spencer Lite Low Fat Chicken, Tomato and Basil (250g/9oz pack).

## Ready-made and Quick and Easy Meals for Vegetarians

● Findus Lean Cuisine Vegetable Tikka Masala (230g/8½oz) pack).
● Marks and Spencer Lite Fresh Vegetable Tikka Masala with Indian Rice.
● Marks and Spencer Fresh Vegetable and Bean Chilli.
● Marks and Spencer Fresh Vegetable Ratatouille.
● Marks and Spencer Filled Red Pepper.

- Marks and Spencer Fresh Vegetable Selection.
- Marks and Spencer Fresh Leek and Mushroom Bake.
- Marks and Spencer Filled Green Pepper.
- Marks and Spencer Fresh Vegetable Ratatouille.
- Marks and Spencer Fresh Vegetable Thai Curry and Rice.
- $\frac{1}{2}$ × 400g (14oz) can Safeway Vegetable Tikka Masala, plus 50g (2oz) (uncooked weight) brown rice.
- $\frac{1}{2}$ × 350g (12oz) tub Safeway Pepper and Basil Pasta Sauce, plus 75g (3oz) (uncooked weight) pasta.
- Sainsbury's Authentic Indian Chobia and Mushroom Bhajee, plus 50g (2oz) (uncooked weight) brown rice.
- Sainsbury's Authentic Indian Chickpea Dhal, plus 50g (2oz) (uncooked weight) brown rice.

## Quick and Easy Cook-in-Sauce Meals

For those with a little more time to cook but who want a quick meal, cook-in-sauces are the answer. They are tasty, easy and can turn an ordinary meal into a banquet – well, almost! I have listed a wide selection here but no doubt you will find plenty more. Check out your local supermarket or store and select any brand that contains 4 per cent or less fat. Follow the cooking instructions on the label, but always adapt them if necessary to avoid cooking with fat or oil of any kind unless you are a vegetarian.

## Low-fat Cooking Method

Chicken, turkey, pork, steak or lamb can all be chopped into bite-sized pieces and dry-fried in a non-stick pan. Once the meat has changed colour, you can add the sauce. If the recipe calls for onions or other vegetables, dry-fry these before you add the sauce.

Choose *one* of the following and add the sauce of your choice. Quantities are per person.

- 175g (6oz) chicken or turkey (weighed without bone), no skin.
- 115 (4oz) red meat, all visible fat removed. If using mince, dry fry and drain away all fat before adding the sauce.
- 225g (8oz) white fish, no skin.

## Cook-in-Sauces

- Asda Sweet and Sour Sauce (serves 4).
- Del Monte Medium Indian with Pineapple and Banana (serves 4).
- Dolmio Light with Mushrooms (serves 4).
- Heinz Weight Watchers Oriental Sweet and Sour Cooking Sauce (serves 3).
- Heinz Weight Watchers Chinese Szechuan Cooking Sauce (serves 3).
- Heinz Weight Watchers French White Wine and Dill Cooking Sauce (serves 3).
- Homepride Low in Fat Creamy Curry Sauce (serves 4).

- Homepride Low in Fat Tomato and Tarragon Sauce (serves 4).
- Homepride Red Wine Sauce (serves 4).
- Homepride Tomato and Onion Sauce (serves 4).
- Ragù Basil and Oregano (serves 4).
- Ragù Red Wine and Herbs (serves 4).
- Uncle Ben's Stir Fry Sweet and Sour Sauce with Crispy Vegetables (serves 4).

## Simple Recipes

Choose between simple and gourmet recipes. Here are the simple ones. The gourmet recipes can be found on pages 165–210.

### Simple Meat Recipes

- Meat Loaf (page 117).
- Sweet and Sour Meatballs (page 117).
- Pork in Savoury Tomato Sauce (page 119).
- Crunchy Bacon and Spaghetti (page 119).
- Gammon and Pineapple Rice (page 120).
- Mixed Bean and Bacon Hotpot (page 121).
- Minced Lamb and Pasta Bake (page 122).
- Moussaka (page 123).
- Stuffed Liver (page 124).

### Simple Poultry Recipes

- Caribbean Chicken (page 125).
- Chicken Cacciatore (page 126).
- Chicken in Chilli and Pepper Sauce (page 127).

- Chicken Herb Parcels (page 127).
- Chicken in Orange and Apricot Sauce (page 128).
- Chicken in Tomato (page 129).
- Chicken Stuffed with Mushrooms and Tarragon (page 130).
- Chilli Chicken and Aubergine Stir-fry (page 131).
- Italian Barbecued Chicken (page 132).
- Middlesex Gumbo (page 133).
- Pineapple Chicken (page 134).
- Spicy Chicken Drumsticks (page 135).
- Chicken or Turkey Tagliatelle with Ginger (page 136).
- Turkey Burgers (page 137).
- Turkey and Pineapple Casserole (page 138).
- Turkey Steaks with Spicy Tomato and Mixed Pepper Sauce (page 139).

## Simple Fish Recipes

- Cidered Lemon Cod Steaks (page 140).
- Cod Parcels (page 141).
- Fish Kebabs (page 142).
- Mackerel Stuffed with Spinach (page 143).
- Mariner's Mediterranean Pie (page 144).
- Stuffed Plaice (page 145).
- Creamy Tuna Pasta (page 146).
- Tuna Fish Pasta (page 147).
- Tuna Rice Bake (page 147).
- Tuna Rice and Peas (page 148).
- Tuna Sauce with Pasta (page 149).
- Tuna and Tarragon Pasta (page 150).

## Simple Vegetarian Recipes

- Bean Pie (page 151).
- Bean and Vegetable Bake (page 152).
- Broccoli Bake (page 153).
- Cauliflower and Courgette Bake (page 154).
- Chickpea Couscous (page 155).
- Flat Stomach Plan Pizza (page 156).
- Hearty Hotpot (page 157).
- Saucy Vegetables and Pasta (page 158).
- Soya Mince and Potato Pie (page 159).
- Spinach and Pasta Bake (page 160).
- Stuffed Marrow (page 161).
- Vegetable Croquettes (page 162).
- Veggie Delight (page 163).
- Wyn's Wonderful Pasta (page 164).

## Gourmet Choices

All these recipes can be used as main course options and some are particularly suited to a dinner party menu.

## Gourmet Meat Recipes

- Barbecued Pork Pouches (page 165).
- Cassoulet (page 167).
- Beef and Mushroom Kebabs (page 167).
- Beef Teriyaki Skewers (page 168).
- Chilli Con Carne (page 169).
- Fillet of Beef with Peppercorns (page 170).
- Hungarian Beef (page 171).

- Spicy Spaghetti Bolognese (page 172).
- Steak and Kidney Pie (page 173).
- Kidney and Tomato Kebabs (page 174).
- Orange and Cranberry Kidneys (page 175).
- Lamb's Liver with Orange (page 176).
- Liver with Red Wine and Rosemary (page 177).

## Gourmet Poultry Recipes

- Chicken in Creamy Apple Sauce (page 178).
- Chicken and Mushroom Pilaff (page 180).
- Chicken and Mushroom Supreme (page 181).
- Chicken à l'Orange (page 182).
- Chicken with Orange and Apricots (page 183).
- Chicken in Orange and Marjoram (page 185).
- Chicken with Paprika and Fennel (page 186).
- Chicken Pilaff (page 187).
- Chicken and Potato Cakes (page 188).
- Chinese Chicken (page 189).
- Glazed Chicken (page 190).
- Hot Chicken Surprise (page 191).

## Gourmet Fish Recipes

- Barbecued Fish Kebabs (page 192).
- Marinated Haddock (page 193).
- Prawn Pilaff (page 194).
- Tagliatelle with Salmon and Scallops (page 195).
- Trout with Herbs (page 196).

## Gourmet Vegetarian Recipes

- Broccoli Gratiné with Cheese and Cannellini Topping (page 197).
- Creamy Horseradish and Watercress Crumble (page 199).
- Egg and Vegetable Sauté (page 200).
- Lentil Roast (page 201).
- Stir-fried Vegetables with Ginger and Sesame Marinade (page 203).
- Three-layer Millet Bake (page 204).
- Tikka Lentil Bake (page 206).
- Tricolour Pasta Risotto (page 208).
- Vegetable Pilaff (page 209).

## Vegetable Accompaniments

The following may be used as accompaniments to any of the main course dishes in this book.

- Dry-roast Parsnips (page 210).
- Dry-roast Potatoes (page 210).
- Lyonnaise Potatoes (page 211).
- Fat-free French Fries (page 211).
- Oven Chips (page 212).
- Potato and Onion Bake (page 213).
- Spicy Potatoes (page 214).
- Lemon-glazed Vegetables (page 215).
- Spinach Roulade with Mushroom Filling (page 216).

# Desserts

*Select any one*

For those of us who have a sweet tooth, it is a real bonus to be able to eat a delectable dessert that is not loaded with calories or fat, and this is invaluable in keeping us on the path to a slimmer and healthier body.

This section offers a variety of flavours and textures. Some of the recipes are child's play to prepare while others are more challenging.

## Quick and Easy Desserts

- 2 pieces any fresh fruit.
- 4 dried apricots soaked overnight in black or fruit tea. Add a pinch of cinnamon to taste and top with 50g (2oz) low-fat fromage frais.
- ½ orange, peeled and sliced, ½ banana, sliced, and 6 grapes, arranged on a plate and served with 50g (2oz) low-fat cottage cheese.
- 1 tablespoon jam mixed with 115g (4oz) low-fat cottage cheese.
- 115g (4oz) canned black cherries in syrup with 60g (2¼oz) Wall's 'Too Good To Be True' ice cream.
- 1 meringue biscuit or meringue nest served or filled with 115g (4oz) fresh fruit of your choice and topped with 50g (2oz) low-fat yogurt or fromage frais.

- 1 meringue nest filled with 25g (1oz) Wall's 'Too Good To Be True' ice cream, plus 50g (2oz) any fresh fruit.
- 1 meringue basket topped with 50g (2oz) Wall's 'Too Good To Be True' double toffee ice cream.
- 2 brown Ryvitas spread with Marmite and topped with 75g (3oz) low-fat cottage cheese.
- 115g (4oz) fresh pineapple rings topped with 1 liqueur glass of Kirsch and served chilled.

## Instant Desserts

- 1 × 150g (5oz) pot Ambrosia Low Fat Rice Pudding.
- 1 pot Asda Very Low Fat Strawberry Tumble.
- 115g (4oz) fresh or stewed fruit served with 150g (5oz) Bird's Low Fat Custard.
- 1 pot Cadbury's Light Low Fat Chocolate Mousse.
- 115g (4oz) Del Monte Sorbet (any flavour).
- 1 pot Marks and Spencer Lite Lemon Mousse.
- 1 pot Marks and Spencer Lite Milk Chocolate Mousse.
- 1 pot Marks and Spencer Summer Fruit Compote.
- 1 pot Marks and Spencer Summer Fruit Pudding, served with 1 teaspoon low-fat fromage frais.
- 1 pot Mullerlight Yogurt (any flavour).
- ½ × 200g (7oz) tub Mullerice Dairy Rice with Caramel, plus 115g (4oz) chopped strawberries.
- ½ × 200g (7oz) tub Mullerice Dairy Rice with Apples in Syrup.

- 1 pot Safeway Virtually Fat Free Yogurt (any flavour).
- 1 pot Reduced Calorie Fruit Cocktail Trifle.
- 1 pot Sainsbury's Low Fat Fool (any flavour).
- 115g (4oz) Sainsbury's Reduced Sugar Supreme Dessert, made up with milk in addition to allowance.
- 1 pot St Ivel Shape Virtually Fat Free Fromage Frais (any flavour).

## Gourmet Desserts

- Apple Jelly with Fromage Frais (page 217).
- Autumn Pudding (page 218).
- Cheese and Apricot Pears (page 219).
- Fresh Fruit Salad (page 219).
- Fruit Crumble (page 220).
- Fruit Delight (page 221).
- Fruit Flan (page 221).
- Ginger and Lemon Fluff (page 222).
- Home-made Ice Cream (page 223).
- Kiwi and Ginger Dessert (page 224).
- Low-fat Trifle (page 225).
- Melon Sundae (page 225).
- Orange and Pineapple Jelly (page 226).
- Peach Melba Jelly Dream (page 226).
- Pineapple Meringue (page 227).
- Pineapple Snow (page 228).
- Strawberry Layer Dessert (page 228).
- Strawberry Sorbet (page 229).
- Strawberry Wine Jelly (page 230).
- Summer Delight (page 231).

- Summer Pudding (page 231).
- Tiramisu (page 233).
- Upside Down Fruit Meringue (page 234).

## Cakes and Loaves

For a change from your usual dessert, try a slice of any of these cakes to eat with your main meal or instead to save as a treat for later in the evening – but not both! While you are on the diet, these should be eaten only as part of your daily food allowance and must not be eaten as an extra. But the good news is, when you reach your goal weight you can have the occasional extra slice as a treat.

For those of you who, like me, find cakes difficult to resist once they are cut into, follow this tip. Allow the cake to cool after cooking, then cut it into slices. Wrap each slice in cling film and freeze in a non-see-through container. You can then take out a slice at a time to defrost as required.

See pages 234–242 for the following recipes.
1 serving = 1 slice as specified.

- Wholemeal Fruit Slice (page 234).
- Apricot Bread (page 235).
- Bran Loaf (page 236).
- Carrot Cake (page 237).
- Carrot and Ginger Cake (page 238).
- Malt Loaf (page 238).
- Marmalade Cake (page 239).

- Moist Fruit Cake (page 240).
- Sultana Loaf (page 241).
- Weetabix Cake (page 241).

# 7
# Recipes

# Breakfasts

## *Austrian Muesli*

SERVES 1

12.5g (½oz) porridge oats
75g (3oz) skimmed or semi-skimmed milk
from allowance
6 sultanas
150g (5oz) natural yogurt
1 teaspoon clear honey

Mix all the ingredients together in a bowl. Cover and place in a refrigerator until morning.

## *Porridge*

SERVES 1

25g (1oz) porridge oats
300ml (½ pint) cold water
25g (1oz) sultanas
liquid sweetener to taste

*to serve*
milk from allowance
1 teaspoon liquid honey

Place the porridge oats and the water in a small saucepan and heat gently until boiling. Add the sultanas and leave to simmer for 5 minutes. Add the liquid sweetener. Leave covered overnight. Stir well and reheat until thoroughly hot.

To serve, pour the milk from your allowance into

a cereal dish, tip the porridge into this and it will float. Now pour on the liquid honey.

## Lunches

### *Bean Salad*

SERVES 2

1 × 200g (7oz) can red kidney beans
1 × 200g (7oz) can cut green beans
1 × 200g (7oz) can chickpeas
1 × 200g (7oz) can butter beans
1 Spanish onion, peeled and chopped
4 tomatoes, chopped
3 sticks celery, washed and finely sliced
75g (3oz) sultanas
150g (5oz) low-fat natural yogurt
salt and black pepper to taste

Drain the beans and chickpeas. Mix with the fresh vegetables and sultanas. Stir in the yogurt and season to taste.

Serve with additional salad vegetables if desired.

# Cheese, Prawn and Asparagus Salad

### SERVES 2

115g (4oz) low-fat cottage cheese
175g (6oz) prawns, cooked and peeled
4 tablespoons chopped and diced cucumber
freshly ground black pepper to taste
unlimited lettuce or watercress
225g (8oz) asparagus tips

Mix the cottage cheese, prawns and cucumber together and season with the pepper.

Lay the mixture on a bed of shredded lettuce or watercress and decorate with the asparagus tips.

# Fruit and Chicken Salad

### SERVES 1

unlimited amounts of shredded lettuce, chopped cucumber and any other green salad items
1 apple, peeled, cored and sliced
1 pear, peeled, cored and sliced
1 orange, peeled and cut into segments
1 kiwi fruit, peeled and sliced
50g (2oz) chicken breast, cooked and chopped
2 tablespoons low-fat natural yogurt
1 tablespoon wine vinegar
1 clove garlic, peeled and crushed
salt and pepper to taste

Arrange the lettuce and salad on a large dinner plate.

Lay the fruit slices and segments on top of the salad and place the chopped chicken in the centre.

Make up a dressing with the yogurt, vinegar and garlic, and season to taste. Serve with the salad.

## Prawn and Pasta Salad

### SERVES 4

450g (1lb) cooked weight, medium-sized pasta shells
450g (1lb) prawns, peeled and cooked
150g (5oz) low-fat natural yogurt
1 tablespoon tomato purée
a few drops of Tabasco sauce to taste
3 spring onions

Combine the cooked pasta shells and prawns in a serving bowl.

In a small bowl, stir together the yogurt, tomato purée and Tabasco sauce. Pour on to the pasta mixture and toss well.

Sprinkle with the spring onions just before serving at room temperature or very slightly chilled.

Serve with a green salad.

# Red Kidney Bean Salad

### SERVES 1

1 × 200g (7oz) can red kidney beans
75g (3oz) peas, cooked
115g (4oz) potatoes, cooked and chopped
chopped mint
150g (5oz) low-fat natural yogurt
green salad vegetables

*to garnish*
onion rings

Drain the kidney beans and mix with the peas, potatoes, mint and yogurt. Serve on a bed of salad vegetables and garnish with onion rings.

# Micro Sandwich

### SERVES 1

2 slices wholemeal bread
1 tablespoon Branston pickle
1 teaspoon mustard
25g (1oz) wafer thin ham
½ fresh onion, thinly sliced
1 tomato, sliced

Spread one slice of bread thinly with the Branston pickle and the other with mustard. Place the ham, onion and tomato on one slice, and place the other slice on top.

Place on a non-metallic plate in the microwave for 1–1½ minutes, on full power.

NB The timing is correct for a 600 watt oven. Adjust the timing according to the wattage of your oven.

# Club Sandwich

SERVES 1

3 slices wholemeal bread
2 Mattessons turkey rashers
tomato ketchup
mustard
HP Fruity Sauce
reduced-oil salad dressing
(any brand)
shredded lettuce
1 tomato, sliced
cucumber slices
25g (1oz) wafer thin chicken

Toast each slice of bread on both sides and grill the turkey rashers until crisp.

Spread 1 slice of toast with tomato ketchup. Spread one side of the second slice with mustard and the other side with HP Fruity Sauce. Spread the third slice with reduced-oil salad dressing.

Place the turkey rashers on top of the first slice of toast and top with shredded lettuce and half the tomato slices. Next, add the second slice of toast, placing it fruity side down. Top with the chicken, cucumber and remaining tomato slices. Place the third slice of toast (spread with reduced-oil salad dressing) on top. Press together firmly and cut into 4 triangles. Secure each triangle with a cocktail stick. Serve while the turkey rashers are still hot.

## Creamy Topping for Baked Potatoes

SERVES 4

450g (16oz) low-fat natural yogurt
chopped parsley
a few spring onions
1 red pepper, diced
salt and pepper to taste

Strain the yogurt through a coffee filter or cloth and leave overnight in the refrigerator to allow the whey to drip through (takes approximately 6 hours to drain).

You will be left with a lovely thick cream cheese substitute. Add the parsley, spring onions, diced pepper, and season with salt and pepper. Use as a topping for baked potatoes.

## Potato and Leek Soup

SERVES 4

3 leeks, washed and sliced
675g (1½lb) potatoes, peeled and sliced
1 litre (1¾ pints) vegetable stock
salt and black pepper to taste
chopped parsley (optional)

Place the leeks in a small amount of water in a large saucepan. Cover with a lid and cook for 10 minutes or until soft.

Add the potatoes (you may need to add a little more liquid) and cook until the vegetables are soft, stirring to prevent them sticking to the pan.

Add the stock and cook for a further 5 minutes.

Allow the soup to cool, then purée with a hand blender or in a food processor.

Season the soup and reheat. Sprinkle with the chopped parsley (if used), and serve, immediately.

NB This is a thick soup, add extra stock if a lighter soup is required.

## *Winter Warmer Soup*

### SERVES 4

2 carrots, sliced
1 onion, peeled and chopped
2 cloves garlic, peeled and crushed
115g (4oz) mushrooms
1 × 225g (8oz) can baked beans
1 × 225g (8oz) can chopped tomatoes
1 tablespoon mixed dried herbs
300ml (½ pint) water
salt and black pepper to taste
4 rashers lean bacon

Place the carrots, onion, garlic and mushrooms in a large non-stick pan and dry-fry until the onion and mushrooms soften, adding a little water, if needed.

Add the beans, tomatoes, mixed herbs and water,

and season with salt and pepper. Bring to the boil and leave to simmer.

Grill the bacon and remove any rind. Cut into small pieces and add to the soup.

Simmer for 30 minutes or until the carrots are soft. Add extra water if required.

Serve immediately with 25g (1oz) crusty bread per person.

# Chicken Drumstick Surprise

### SERVES 4

25g (1oz) breadcrumbs
1 teaspoon dried rosemary
1 teaspoon dried thyme
1 teaspoon dried oregano
1 clove garlic, peeled and crushed
salt and black pepper to taste
4 chicken drumsticks
2 tablespoons low-fat natural yogurt

Place all the ingredients in a bag and shake to mix together.

Using a sharp knife cut slits in the drumsticks and coat with the yogurt. Place the drumsticks in the bag and coat with the dry ingredients.

Cook the coated drumsticks under a preheated grill for 15 minutes, turning them once. To check if the chicken is cooked, insert a sharp knife into the flesh. If the juices are pink, continue cooking for a further 5 minutes.

Serve with a green salad.

# Baked Potatoes with Apple

### SERVES 4

4 large baking potatoes
½ medium cooking apple
1 large onion, peeled and finely chopped
1 teaspoon dried sage
½ teaspoon mustard powder
salt to taste

Preheat the oven to 200°C, 400°F or Gas mark 6.

Wash and prick the potatoes, sprinkle with salt and cook in the oven for 1½ hours.

Remove the potatoes from the oven and allow to cool for a while. Cut the potatoes in half and scoop out the middles into a bowl, leaving the skins intact, and mash the potato well.

Peel, core and finely chop the apple. Dry-fry the onion in a non-stick frying pan until the onion begins to soften. Stir in the apple and cook for a further 2–4 minutes until soft.

Add the onion and apple mixture to the mashed potato. Add the sage, mustard and salt and mix thoroughly.

Spoon the mixture back into the potato skins and return to the oven for a further 15 minutes or until the tops are browned.

Serve with salad.

# Smoked Haddock and Potato Boats

### SERVES 4

4 large baking potatoes
2 tablespoons virtually fat-free fromage frais
salt and freshly ground black pepper to taste
115g (4oz) smoked haddock, cooked and flaked

*to garnish*
fresh parsley

Preheat the oven to 180°C, 350°F or Gas mark 4.

Wash and prick the potatoes and bake in the oven for 1½–2 hours.

When soft, cut each potato in half lengthwise. Leaving the skins intact, scoop the insides of each potato half into a bowl. Add the fromage frais, salt and pepper, and mash well.

Stir in the smoked haddock and spoon the mixture back into the potato skins. Turn the oven up to 200°C, 400°F or Gas mark 6. Return the potatoes to the oven for a further 10–15 minutes.

Sprinkle with the parsley and serve immediately with salad.

# Dinners

## STARTERS

### *Cucumber Boats with Tuna*

SERVES 4

1 cucumber
whites of 2 hard-boiled eggs
225g (8oz) can of tuna in brine
115g (4oz) quark or other low-fat soft cheese or
cottage cheese
1 teaspoon made-up mustard
1 tablespoon lemon juice
1 tablespoon chopped parsley
1 tablespoon chopped chives or spring onions
salt and pepper to taste
a few lettuce leaves

Peel the cucumber, cut off the ends and cut in half.
Then slice each half in two lengthways. Remove the
seeds with a ball-cutter or teaspoon and discard.
Blanch the cucumber shells in boiling salted water
for 3–5 minutes. Drain and chill under cold running
water. Pat dry with kitchen paper.

Chop the egg whites and place to one side.

Drain the tuna and, using a fork, mash together
with the quark, soft cheese or cottage cheese and the
mustard and lemon juice. If you prefer a smoother
mixture, purée the fish and other ingredients in a
food processor or liquidiser. Stir in most of the
parsley and chives or spring onions and season to
taste.

Fill the cucumber shells with the mixture and arrange on a lettuce-covered dish or individual plates. Sprinkle the chopped egg whites and remaining herbs over the top.

Chill in the refrigerator until required.

## Garlic Mushrooms

### SERVES 4

450g (1lb) button mushrooms
300ml (½ pint) chicken stock
3 cloves of fresh garlic, peeled and finely sliced
salt and pepper to taste

Wash the mushrooms and drain. Place the chicken stock and garlic in a saucepan. Bring to the boil and simmer for 5 minutes on a gentle heat. Add the mushrooms, cover the saucepan with a lid and simmer for a further 7 minutes. Season to taste before serving.

Serve in individual soup dishes and eat with a spoon.

# *Low-fat Hummus with Crudités*

## SERVES 2

115g (4oz) chickpeas, pre-soaked in cold water
overnight
7 tablespoons skimmed milk in addition to
allowance
1 tablespoon lemon juice
½ teaspoon mild chilli powder
¼ teaspoon garlic granules
¼ teaspoon ground white pepper
salt
2 tablespoons low-fat natural yogurt

*for the crudités*

red pepper
cucumber
celery
cauliflower florets
⎫
⎬ all cut into sticks
⎭

Drain the chickpeas and place in a saucepan. Cover
with fresh water and bring to the boil. Reduce the
heat, cover and simmer gently for 2–2¼ hours until
the chickpeas are soft. Drain.

Place the chickpeas, skimmed milk and lemon
juice in a food processor or liquidiser and blend on
high speed until the mixture is pale and smooth.
Stir into this the chilli powder, garlic granules, white
pepper, salt and yogurt.

Spoon into a serving dish and chill before serving.

Serve with the raw vegetable sticks and cauliflower
florets.

# *Melon Salad*

SERVES 4

1 honeydew melon
450g (1lb) tomatoes
1 large cucumber
salt
1 tablespoon parsley
Oil-free Vinaigrette Dressing (see recipe, page 243)
1 heaped teaspoon chopped mint and chives

Cut the melon in half, remove the seeds and scoop out the flesh. A curved grapefruit knife is useful for this. Cut the flesh into cubes.

Skin and quarter the tomatoes, squeeze out the seeds and remove the core. Cut into quarters again if the tomatoes are large.

Peel the cucumber and cut into small cubes about the same size as the melon cubes. Sprinkle with salt, cover with a plate and stand for 30 minutes. Drain away the liquid and rinse the cubes in cold water.

Mix the fruit and the vegetables together in a deep bowl. Pour the dressing over them, cover and chill for 2–3 hours.

Just before serving, mix in the herbs.

As this salad makes a lot of juice it is easier to eat with a spoon.

# Prawn or Crab Cocktail

## SERVES 4

4 tablespoons tomato sauce
3 tablespoons low-fat salad cream
225g (8oz) prawns, shelled and cooked or 1 × 225g
(8oz) can crabmeat, drained
1 crisp eating apple, peeled and chopped
lettuce
paprika

*to garnish*
4 slices lime or lemon

Mix the tomato sauce and salad cream together.

Mix together the prawns or crab and apple, and add the sauce.

Shred the lettuce and place in 4 individual dishes. Spoon the cocktail mixture into the dishes, and chill.

Just before serving, sprinkle with paprika and garnish each dish with a twist of lime or lemon.

# Smoked Mackerel Pâté

## SERVES 6

115g (4oz) smoked mackerel
225g (8oz) low-fat cottage cheese
1–2 teaspoons horseradish sauce
2 teaspoons lemon juice
salt and white pepper to taste

Skin the mackerel and remove any bones, then break it into medium-sized pieces.

Place the mackerel and all the remaining ingredients in a food processor or liquidiser and purée until smooth.

Taste and add more horseradish sauce, lemon juice, salt and pepper if desired. Turn out into a dish. Cover and chill until required.

Serve with 1 slice toast (no butter) per person.

# Cream of Courgette Soup

## SERVES 4

You will find this soup has a surprisingly smooth and delicate taste.

4 medium courgettes
600ml (1 pint) beef stock
salt and pepper to taste

Peel the courgettes and cut into thick slices. Place them in a large saucepan and cover with the stock. Cook on a medium heat until the courgettes are soft.

Once the courgettes are cooked, place the mixture in a food processor or liquidiser and blend until smooth. Season to taste with a little salt and pepper and serve. Maintenance dieters can add a single portion of Dairylea Light into the soup and let it melt before serving.

# Fresh Vegetable Soup

## SERVES 4

2 large carrots, chopped
1 large potato, peeled and chopped
115g (4oz) cabbage, shredded
50g (2oz) peas
50g (2oz) sweetcorn (optional)
1 large onion, peeled and chopped
1–2 litres (2 pints) water
1 vegetable stock cube
freshly ground black pepper to taste

Place all the vegetables in a large saucepan with the water. Cover and bring to the boil. Add the stock cube and simmer for 1 hour. Add a generous sprinkling of black pepper to taste. Allow to cool, then place in a food processor or liquidiser on high speed for 15 seconds.

Store in the refrigerator until needed.

# Gazpacho

## SERVES 2

1 large Spanish onion, peeled and chopped
1 small can chopped tomatoes
1 clove garlic, peeled and crushed (more if desired)
300ml (½ pint) cold water
1 teaspoon dried mixed herbs
salt and black pepper to taste
½ red pepper, deseeded and cut into squares
½ green pepper, deseeded and cut into squares

*to garnish*
extra chopped mixed herbs

Place the onion, half the chopped tomatoes, the garlic, water, herbs and seasoning in a food processor. Process until the mixture is of a fairly smooth consistency. Pour into a serving bowl.

Add the pepper and remaining tomatoes. Add a few ice cubes and chill in the refrigerator for about half an hour.

Garnish with the herbs and serve.

# Low-fat Creamy Potato and Parsley Soup

### SERVES 2

4 medium-sized potatoes
150ml (¼ pint) water
300ml (½ pint) skimmed or virtually fat-free milk in addition to allowance
4 tablespoons virtually fat-free fromage frais
¼ tablespoon chopped parsley
salt and black pepper to taste.

Peel and cut the potatoes into quarters and place in a saucepan with water. Bring to the boil and cook until firm but soft in the middle. Drain, reserving the water.

Place the milk and potato water in a separate saucepan and heat gently. Add the fromage frais and stir.

Add the cooked potatoes, remove from the heat

and blend with a hand blender until most of the potatoes have liquidised, but some 'lumps' are left to give texture.

Stir in the parsley, salt and pepper and reheat gently but do not boil. Serve immediately.

## Pea and Lettuce Soup
### SERVES 4

2 onions, peeled and chopped
$\frac{1}{4}$–$\frac{1}{2}$ cup chopped mint
2–3 cups shredded lettuce (outside leaves)
450g (1lb) frozen peas
1.2 litres (2 pints) water
2 chicken stock cubes
salt and pepper to taste

Cook the onion and mint in a little water in a saucepan until soft.

Add the shredded lettuce, peas, water and stock cubes. Season with salt and pepper and simmer for 10 minutes uncovered.

Place in a food processor or liquidiser and process until smooth. Taste and adjust the seasoning, if necessary.

Serve immediately.

## MAIN COURSES:

## SIMPLE MEAT RECIPES

# Meat Loaf

### SERVES 6

675g (1½lb) lean minced beef
1 cup porridge oats
225g (8oz) carrot, grated
1 large onion, grated or finely chopped
1 teaspoon horseradish sauce
1 teaspoon Worcester sauce
salt and pepper to taste
1 egg (to bind)

Preheat the oven to 180°C, 350°F or Gas mark 4.
Line a 900g (2lb) loaf tin with foil.
Place all the ingredients in a bowl and mix thoroughly with your hands. Place the mixture in the loaf tin and cook in the oven for 1½ hours.
Serve with jacket potatoes and mixed salad.

# Sweet and Sour Meatballs

### SERVES 4

*for the meatballs*
450g (1lb) beef, turkey, pork or lamb
1 egg (to bind)
1 cup breadcrumbs
pinch of salt
1 onion, peeled and grated

*for the sauce*
75g (3oz) brown sugar
3 level teaspoons cornflour
7 tablespoons water
4 tablespoons vinegar
1 vegetable stock cube
1 small can pineapple pieces (plus juice)
1 tablespoon soy sauce

Mix together all the meatball ingredients. Carefully shape the mixture into small meatballs and press well together.

Place the meatballs under a preheated grill and cook gently for 15 minutes, turning them regularly to ensure even cooking.

To make the sauce, mix the brown sugar and cornflour together in a saucepan. Blend in the water, vinegar, stock cube, pineapple juice and soy sauce. Cook and stir until thick and bubbly. Stir in the meatballs and pineapple pieces, and simmer very gently for 15 minutes.

Serve with rice or noodles (50g/2oz uncooked weight per person) and stir-fried vegetables.

# Pork in Savoury Tomato Sauce

### SERVES 2

2 × 115g (2 × 4oz) lean pork steaks
1 small can chopped tomatoes
1 onion, peeled and chopped
115g (4oz) mushrooms, washed and chopped
1 teaspoon mixed dried herbs
1 vegetable stock cube

Preheat the oven to 190°C, 375°F or Gas mark 5.

Dry-fry the pork to seal the juices. Place in a casserole dish, add the tomatoes, onion, mushrooms, herbs and stock cube.

Place the lid on the casserole dish and bake in the oven for 1 hour.

Serve with new or Dry-roast Potatoes (see recipe, pages 210–11) and vegetables.

# Crunchy Bacon and Spaghetti

### SERVES 1

3 thin slices lean smoked bacon
50g (2oz) uncooked weight wholemeal spaghetti
1 small can of chopped tomatoes
2 medium-sized mushrooms, thinly sliced
2 tablespoons frozen sweetcorn
1 tablespoon Branston pickle
2 teaspoons cornflour
salt and pepper to taste

Trim any fat from the bacon and grill on both sides.

Cook the spaghetti in boiling water for 10 minutes.

While the spaghetti is cooking empty the tomatoes into a saucepan and add the mushrooms, sweetcorn and pickle. Cook on a moderate heat, then allow to simmer.

Wipe off any traces of fat from the bacon, using kitchen paper, then snip into bite-size pieces and add to the tomato mixture.

Dissolve the cornflour in cold water and add gradually to the tomato mixture to thicken it as it simmers. Season to taste.

By the time the spaghetti is cooked the bacon and tomato mixture will be ready to serve. Drain the spaghetti, place on a serving plate and top with the bacon and tomato mixture.

# Gammon and Pineapple Rice

### SERVES 1

1 gammon steak
1 small onion, peeled and finely chopped
1 small can pineapple chunks (plus juice)
$\frac{1}{2}$ vegetable stock cube
150ml ($\frac{1}{4}$ pint) water
50g (2oz) (uncooked weight) rice
50g (2oz) peas, canned or frozen
$\frac{1}{2}$ red pepper, sliced
dash of soy sauce
salt and pepper to taste

Cut the gammon steak into cubes and gently dry-fry with the onion in a non-stick pan.

Add the pineapple and juice, stock cube, water and rice, bring to the boil, cover and cook for 10 minutes or until the rice is tender and most of the liquid is absorbed. If necessary, add more boiling water during cooking.

Add the peas, red pepper and soy sauce and season with salt and pepper.

Heat through and serve.

# Mixed Bean and Bacon Hotpot

SERVES 3

3 baking potatoes
2 rashers smoked lean bacon, chopped
1 large onion, peeled and chopped
1 small can red kidney beans
1 small can baked beans
1 small can chopped tomatoes

Preheat the oven to 200°C, 400°F or Gas mark 6.

Wash and dry the potatoes. Prick the skins and rub with salt. Cook in the oven for 1½ hours.

Dry-fry the bacon and onion in a non-stick pan. Drain the kidney beans and add to the pan. Add all the remaining ingredients, bring to the boil and simmer for 20–25 minutes.

Serve with jacket potatoes.

# Minced Lamb and Pasta Bake

## SERVES 6

450g (1lb) minced lamb
1 onion, peeled and chopped
1 clove garlic, peeled and crushed
150ml (¼ pint) water
1 × 400g (14oz) can tomatoes
1 tablespoon tomato purée
a dash of Worcester sauce
1 tablespoon fresh basil
salt and pepper to taste
175g (6oz) (uncooked weight) macaroni
or pasta shapes
300ml (½ pint) semi-skimmed milk in
addition to allowance
1 level teaspoon cornflour
1 teaspoon mustard

Preheat the oven to 180°C, 350°F or Gas mark 4.

Dry-fry the minced lamp in a non-stick pan. Remove from the pan and drain through a sieve or colander, to remove the fat.

Dry-fry the onion and garlic in the pan until soft.

Return the mince to the pan. Add the onion, garlic and water. Cook for 5 minutes.

Add the tomatoes, tomato purée, Worcester sauce, basil, salt and pepper, and simmer for 10–15 minutes.

Meanwhile, boil the pasta according to the instructions on the packet. When cooked, drain and put to one side.

Mix 2 teaspoons of the milk with the cornflour. Heat the remaining milk in a saucepan and, when nearly boiling, add the cornflour mixture, and stir continuously until thickened. Add the mustard, and season to taste.

Add the cooked pasta to the pan with the meat mixture and stir.

Arrange the lamb and pasta mixture in the bottom of an ovenproof dish and top with the milk sauce. Bake in the oven for approximately 20 minutes.

Serve with salad.

# Moussaka

### SERVES 4

2 medium aubergines
450g (1lb) lean minced lamb or beef
1 medium onion, peeled and sliced
2 cloves garlic, peeled and crushed
4 tablespoons tomato purée
1 teaspoon mixed dried herbs
1 teaspoon ground cinnamon
salt and black pepper to taste

*for the topping*
2 eggs
1 level tablespoon cornflour
salt and black pepper to taste
225g (8oz) low-fat natural yogurt
½ teaspoon nutmeg

Preheat the oven to 180°C, 350°F or Gas mark 4.

Cut the aubergines into ½cm (¼in) slices and sprinkle with salt. Leave for 30 minutes.

Dry-fry the minced lamb or beef in a non-stick pan for a few minutes. Remove from the pan and drain away the excess fat. Return the mince to the pan. Add the onions and dry-fry for 5 minutes until transparent. Add the garlic and cook for 2 minutes. Add the tomato purée, mixed herbs, cinnamon and seasoning and simmer for 15 minutes.

Rinse the aubergine slices in cold water and pat dry on kitchen paper.

Lightly grease an ovenproof dish and arrange one layer of aubergine to cover the base. Spread the meat mixture on top and finish with a layer of aubergine.

Beat the eggs, then blend in the cornflour, salt and pepper and whisk in the yogurt. Pour over the aubergine mixture, sprinkle with nutmeg and bake for about 1 hour until the aubergines are tender and the top is golden.

## Stuffed Liver

### SERVES 2

225g (8oz) pig's or lamb's liver, sliced
1 × 400g (14oz) can tomatoes
1 teaspoon sugar
salt and pepper to taste
2 rashers of back bacon with fat cut off
50g (2oz) stuffing mix made up

Preheat the oven to 180°C, 350°F or Gas mark 4.

Wash the liver in cold water and place in the base of an ovenproof dish.

Mix together the tomatoes, sugar, salt and pepper and pour the mixture over the liver.

Arrange the bacon on top of the tomatoes and spread the stuffing mixture on top.

Cook in the oven for 1 hour.

Remove from the oven and place under the grill to crisp the bacon.

Serve immediately with green vegetables.

## MAIN COURSES:

## SIMPLE POULTRY RECIPES

# Caribbean Chicken

### SERVES 2

1 small can pineapple chunks in natural juice
1 large banana, chopped
juice of 1 lemon or lime
2 chicken breasts, skinned
1 small onion, peeled and finely chopped
1 teaspoon brown sugar
1 clove garlic, peeled and crushed
2 teaspoons curry powder or paste (mild)
½ teaspoon allspice
few drops of Tabasco
½ red pepper, diced
300ml (½ pint) chicken stock
salt and pepper to taste

Place the pineapple (and juice) and banana in a bowl. Add the lemon or lime juice.

Dry-fry the chicken for 3–5 mins in a non-stick pan until brown. Remove from the pan.

Add the onion to the pan and dry-fry until it starts to brown. Add the brown sugar and stir well.

Add the garlic and heat gently for a few minutes, then add the curry powder or paste, allspice, Tabasco and red pepper.

Return the chicken to the pan. Add the chicken stock and the pineapple and banana mixture. Simmer gently for 15 minutes and season to taste.

Serve on a bed of boiled brown rice (50g/2oz uncooked weight per person).

# Chicken Cacciatore

### SERVES 4

1 medium onion, peeled and cut into rings
225g (8oz) mushrooms, chopped
1 red pepper, deseeded and cut into strips
2 cloves garlic, peeled and crushed
4 chicken breasts, skinned and cut into cubes
150ml (¼ pint) red wine
2 teaspoons fresh basil
2 teaspoons fresh oregano
1 × 400g (14oz) can chopped tomatoes with herbs
salt and pepper to taste

Dry-fry the onion, mushrooms and red pepper in a non-stick pan. And the garlic and cook until slightly brown.

Add the chicken, wine, herbs, tomatoes and seasoning. Cover and simmer for 40 minutes.

Serve with unlimited vegetables.

# Chicken in Chilli and Pepper Sauce

## SERVES 2

2 chillis (or to taste), sliced
2–3 cloves of garlic, peeled and sliced
2 chicken breast fillets, skinned and cut into cubes
1 × 400g (14oz) can tomatoes
2 teaspoons soft brown sugar
2 teaspoons tomato purée
1 red pepper, sliced
1 green pepper, sliced
salt and pepper to taste

Gently cook the chillis and garlic in a non-stick frying pan with a little water until softened.

Add the chicken and dry-fry to seal it, then add the tomatoes and sugar and stir well. Cook for 5 minutes.

Add the tomato purée, mix well, then add the sliced peppers. Simmer for approximately 30 minutes, stirring occasionally.

Season to taste and serve with boiled tagliatelle (or any pasta) or rice (50g/2oz uncooked weight per person).

# Chicken Herb Parcels

## SERVES 4

4 chicken breast fillets
1 tablespoon fresh coriander
grated rind and juice of 1 orange
2 cloves garlic, peeled and crushed (optional)

Preheat the oven to 190°C, 375°F or Gas mark 5.

Skin the chicken breasts and pat dry with kitchen paper. Slice each chicken breast almost in half and lay out flat.

Sprinkle one half of each breast with the coriander, and sprinkle the other halves with the grated orange rind. Divide the garlic (if used) between the chicken breasts.

Fold over the other half of each chicken breast, place in an ovenproof dish lined with foil, making sure you have enough foil to fold over. Pour the juice from the orange over the chicken and fold the foil over until well sealed.

Bake in the oven for approximately 45 minutes until cooked.

Serve with boiled rice (50g/2oz uncooked weight per person).

## Chicken in Orange and Apricot Sauce

### SERVES 4

300ml (½ pint) orange juice
150ml (¼ pint) apple juice
2 tablespoons lemon juice
1 medium onion, peeled and sliced
2 tablespoons freshly grated root ginger
12 dried apricots, halved
8 chicken thighs, skinned

Mix together all the ingredients, except the chicken,

in a large microwave-safe dish. Add the chicken, cover and microwave on high for 5 minutes. Stir well. Place the dish back in the microwave and cook on medium for 10 minutes, stirring halfway through.

Remove the chicken from the sauce and place in a hot serving dish. Cover and set aside. Return the sauce to the microwave and cook on high for 5 minutes to reduce the liquid. Pour the sauce over the chicken and serve.

NB Timings are correct for a 700 watt oven. Adjust if necessary according to the wattage of your oven.

Alternatively the chicken and sauce can be cooked in a saucepan for 25–30 minutes or casseroled in the oven for 30–40 minutes at 190°C, 375°F or Gas mark 5.

## Chicken in Tomato

### SERVES 4

8 chicken thighs, skinned
1 onion, peeled and sliced
2 carrots, sliced
2 large mushrooms, chopped
salt and pepper to taste
1 level teaspoon mixed herbs.
1 small can Campbell's condensed tomato soup

Preheat the oven to 150°C, 325°F or Gas mark 3.

Place the chicken, onion, carrots and mushrooms in an ovenproof casserole dish. Sprinkle the salt, pepper and mixed herbs over the casserole mixture.

Pour the soup over, cover and bake in the oven until the chicken is cooked through. (Do not make the soup up to the full amount by adding water as the sauce will be too thin.)

Serve with jacket potatoes, rice or pasta (50g/2oz uncooked weight per person) and green vegetables.

# Chicken Stuffed with Mushrooms and Tarragon

### SERVES 2

2 chicken breasts, boned and skinned
115g (4oz) mushrooms, finely chopped
$\frac{1}{2}$ teaspoon dried tarragon
1 tablespoon dried tomatoes
2 tablespoons clear honey
grated rind and juice of 1 large or 2 small limes

Preheat the oven to 200°C, 400°F or Gas mark 6.

Flatten the chicken with a steak mallet.

Mix together the mushrooms, tarragon and tomatoes. Place half the mixture on the centre of each chicken breast. Roll up and secure with cocktail sticks.

Heat a non-stick pan and when quite hot add the chicken and cook until brown and sealed all over. Transfer the chicken and sauce to an ovenproof dish.

Mix together the honey, grated rind and lime juice and pour over the chicken. Cover with foil and bake in the oven for 15 minutes. Remove the foil and bake for a further 15 minutes, basting twice.

Serve with new potatoes and green vegetables.

# Chilli Chicken and Aubergine Stir-fry

## SERVES 3-4

1 aubergine
1 head of fresh broccoli
1 packet noodles (3 layers)
250g (9oz) chicken breast fillets, skinned
1 large onion, peeled and cut into chunks
1 red pepper, cut into large squares
1 yellow pepper, cut into large squares
1 large carrot, cut into julienne strips
2 cloves garlic, peeled and crushed
$\frac{1}{4}$ cup light soy sauce
225g (8oz) fresh mushrooms
$\frac{1}{2}$ bottle oyster sauce
2 teaspoons hot chilli sauce
1 chicken stock cube

Chop the aubergine into large squares. Sprinkle with salt, leave for 15 minutes, then rinse and dry. Steam for 5–10 minutes or boil until soft but not mushy.

Cut the broccoli into florets and steam for 3–5 minutes or microwave for 2 minutes until slightly cooked but still firm.

Place the noodles in a bowl of boiling water, cover and leave for 4 minutes, then drain.

Cut the chicken into thin strips. Heat a large non-stick frying pan and dry-fry the strips of chicken until cooked and browned. Remove and keep warm.

Place the onion, peppers, carrot, garlic and soy sauce in the pan and stir-fry for approximately 2 minutes. Add the mushrooms and broccoli and stir-fry for a further minute.

Add the chicken and aubergine followed by the oyster and chilli sauce. Heat through, then add the cooked noodles and stock cube. Taste and add more chilli sauce if you prefer it hotter. Add water if the mixture begins to stick.

Mix all the ingredients thoroughly and serve.

## Italian Barbecued Chicken

### SERVES 4

1 small can chopped tomatoes
1 small onion, peeled and finely chopped
1 small chilli, finely chopped
4 gloves garlic, peeled and crushed
2 teaspoons dried oregano
2 drops Tabasco sauce
1 teaspoon Worcester sauce
pinch of salt and pepper
1 teaspoon sugar
4 × 175g (4 × 6oz) chicken breasts, skinned

Mix together all the ingredients, except the chicken, in a bowl and brush over the chicken.

Place the coated chicken breasts under a hot grill or on a barbecue and cook thoroughly, turning frequently to ensure even cooking.

Serve with salad.

# *Middlesex Gumbo*

### SERVES 6

1 medium onion, peeled and chopped
1 green pepper, chopped
2 sticks celery, sliced
1 × 400g (14oz) can tomatoes
1½ tablespoons plain flour
½ teaspoon dried thyme
750ml (1¼ pints) water
2 chicken stock cubes
1 small bay leaf
225g (8oz) fresh okra (ladies' fingers)
500g (1¼lb) cooked diced chicken
½ teaspoon salt
½ teaspoon ground pepper

Spray a saucepan with a low-fat spray and cook the onion on a medium heat.

Add the green pepper and celery and cook for about 5 minutes, stirring occasionally. Add the tomatoes.

Blend in the flour and thyme.

Gradually add the water, stock cubes and the bay leaf and cook, stirring occasionally, until the mixture comes to the boil. Reduce the heat and simmer for 1 hour.

Wipe and trim the okra. Add the okra and chicken to the pan and simmer for 10 minutes. Season to taste.

Serve on a bed of boiled brown rice (50g/2oz uncooked weight per person).

# *Pineapple Chicken*

### SERVES 4

4 medium-sized chicken breasts, skinned
1 large can pineapple rings in natural juice
1 onion, sliced
½ teaspoon ground ginger
½ teaspoon dried rosemary
1 level tablespoon cornflour

Preheat the oven to 180°C, 350°F or Gas mark 4.

Place the chicken breasts in an ovenproof dish. Drain the pineapple rings, reserving the juice. Lay the pineapple slices and onion rings over the chicken. Sprinkle the ground ginger and rosemary over.

Mix the pineapple juice with the cornflour and pour over the casserole ingredients.

Cook in the oven for 45 minutes until the chicken is tender.

Serve with boiled brown rice (50g/2oz uncooked weight per person) and salad or new potatoes and vegetables.

# Spicy Chicken Drumsticks

### SERVES 6

115g (4oz) dried breadcrumbs
115g (4oz) wholemeal plain flour
½ teaspoon garlic granules
½ freshly ground black pepper
½ teaspoon dried thyme
½ teaspoon dried basil
¼ teaspoon cayenne pepper
½ teaspoon dried oregano
6 chicken drumsticks, skinned
150g (5oz) low-fat natural yogurt

Preheat the oven to 200°C, 400°F or Gas mark 6.

Place all the dry ingredients in a strong plastic bag and shake well to mix thoroughly.

Dip each chicken drumstick thoroughly in the yogurt, then toss each one, one at a time, in the breadcrumb mixture in the plastic bag to coat thoroughly.

Place the coated drumsticks on a non-stick baking sheet and bake in the oven for 1 hour or until brown and crispy, turning every 15 minutes to ensure even cooking.

Serve with Fat-free French Fries (see recipe, pages 211–12) and mixed salad.

# Chicken or Turkey Tagliatelle with Ginger

### SERVES 4

4 rashers lean smoked bacon, trimmed
4 chicken or turkey breasts, skinned and cubed
1 onion, peeled and chopped
225g (8oz) mushrooms
root ginger (approximately 2–5cm/1–2in square),
peeled and finely grated
1 medium-sized jar of traditional Ragù
225g (8oz) egg-free tagliatelle, preferably white and
green varieties
2 tablespoons low-fat natural yogurt

Chop the bacon into small squares and dry-fry. Add
the chicken or turkey and dry-fry for 5 minutes.
Add the onion and mushrooms to the pan and dry-
fry. Add the root ginger and cook for 2 minutes than
add the Ragù. Stir and heat through. Put a lid on the
saucepan to keep the sauce warm while you prepare
the tagliatelle.

Cook the tagliatelle as directed on the packet and
drain.

Just before serving, mix in the yogurt to either the
sauce or the drained tagliatelle for a creamy effect.

Serve the sauce on the bed of tagliatelle.

# Turkey Burgers

SERVES 4

450g (1lb) lean minced turkey
1 small onion, finely chopped
115g (4oz) wholemeal breadcrumbs made from 3
slices bread
1 teaspoon dried thyme
2 egg whites
salt and pepper to taste
flour for dusting

Place all the ingredients except the flour in a large bowl and mix thoroughly.

Take a handful of the mixture at a time and shape into burgers. The mixture should make 12–16 burgers.

Cover the burgers with a dusting of flour and place in the refrigerator to chill for 15 minutes.

Place the burgers under a preheated grill and cook for about 15–20 minutes, turning once.

Serve with Fat-free French Fries (see recipe, pages 211–12) and a green salad.

Lean minced beef can be substituted for turkey in this recipe.

# Turkey and Pineapple Casserole

### SERVES 2

2 × 175g (2 × 6oz) turkey breast fillets, skinned
1 green pepper, chopped
1 onion, peeled and chopped
1 small can pineapple chunks in natural juice
1 teaspoon curry powder
25g (1oz) cornflour
1 tablespoon tomato ketchup
300ml (½ pint) chicken stock

Preheat the oven to 180°C, 350°F or Gas mark 4.

In a non-stick pan, dry-fry the turkey until brown. Add the green pepper and onion and dry-fry gently for five minutes. Place in a casserole dish. Drain the pineapple chunks, reserving the juice. Add the pineapple chunks to the casserole.

In a saucepan mix 2 tablespoons of the pineapple juice with the curry powder, cornflour and tomato ketchup. Add the chicken stock to the mixture and heat gently, stirring continuously to thicken the liquid. Pour into the casserole and bake in the oven for approximately 1 hour or until cooked.

Serve with boiled brown rice (50g/2oz uncooked weight per person) or new or baked potatoes and salad or vegetables.

# Turkey Steaks with Spicy Tomato and Mixed Pepper Sauce

### SERVES 4

4 turkey steaks
1 onion, peeled and sliced
½ green pepper, shredded
½ red pepper, shredded
½ yellow pepper, shredded
1 × 400g (14oz) can chopped tomatoes
1 tablespoon Worcester sauce
2 teaspoons caster sugar
salt and pepper to taste
1 teaspoon cornflour

Preheat the oven to 180°C, 350°F or Gas mark 4.

Place the steaks in an ovenproof casserole.

In a non-stick saucepan dry-fry the onion and peppers gently for 5 minutes, shaking the pan occasionally. Stir in the tomatoes, Worcester sauce, sugar, salt and pepper.

Blend the cornflour with a little water then add to the pan, stirring continually while bringing to the boil. Pour over the steaks, cover the casserole with a lid or foil and bake in the centre of the oven for 1 hour.

## MAIN COURSES:

### SIMPLE FISH RECIPES

# *Cidered Lemon Cod Steaks*

SERVES 4

4 cod steaks
150ml (¼ pint) medium sweet cider
2 tablespoons orange juice
1 clove garlic, peeled and crushed
2 teaspoons light soy sauce
4 spring onions, trimmed and chopped
salt and pepper to taste
225g (8oz) courgettes, sliced
3 leeks, trimmed and sliced
2 teaspoons grated lemon rind

*to garnish*
2 lemons, cut into quarters
fresh dill

Preheat the oven to 190°C, 375°F or Gas mark 5.

Place the cod steaks in a shallow ovenproof dish.

Mix together the cider, orange juice, garlic, soy sauce, most of the spring onions and seasoning, and pour over the cod steaks. Cover and place in the refrigerator to marinate for 1 hour, turning once or twice. After marinating, bake in the oven for 30–40 minutes.

Lightly cook the courgettes, leeks and lemon rind in a little water for a few minutes until just tender. Season to taste.

Remove the cod from the oven and arrange on a

serving plate. Top with the reserved spring onions and surround with the vegetables and a little sauce.

Garnish with the lemon quarters and fresh dill and serve immediately.

## Cod Parcels

SERVES 4

4 cod fillets
1 onion, peeled and chopped
1 green pepper, deseeded and chopped
fresh parsley, chopped
salt and pepper to taste
1 × 150g (5oz) carton low-fat natural yogurt
1 level teaspoon cornflour

Preheat the oven to 190°C, 375°F or Gas mark 5.

Skin the fish fillets and lay each in the centre of a sheet of greaseproof paper.

Place the onion and pepper on a plate or dish and soften in the microwave for approximately 4–5 minutes on high, or dry-fry until soft if preferred.

Divide the onion and pepper equally and place on top of each fish fillet. Sprinkle with chopped parsley and season with salt and pepper.

Mix the yogurt with the cornflour and place a tablespoon of yogurt on top of each fillet of fish. Fold over the greaseproof paper and tuck in the edges to make 4 parcels.

Place the parcels in an ovenproof dish and cook in the oven for approximately 10–15 minutes.

Remove the fish from the greaseproof paper and serve with boiled new potatoes and peas or a green salad.

## Fish Kebabs

### SERVES 4

225g (8oz) cod fillet, skinned and cut into 2.5cm (1in) chunks
225g (8oz) salmon steak, skinned and cut into 2.5cm (1in) chunks
1 red onion, peeled and cut into 8 pieces
1 green pepper, deseeded and cut into 12 chunks
grated rind and juice of 2 limes
1 tablespoon soy sauce
1 tablespoon white wine vinegar
150ml (¼ pint) dry white wine
salt and pepper to taste

Thread alternate pieces of cod, salmon, onion and pepper on to skewers and place on a shallow dish.

Mix together the lime rind and juice, soy sauce, vinegar, wine and seasoning. Pour over the kebabs.

Cover the kebabs and leave to marinate in the refrigerator for 1 hour, turning at least once.

Preheat the grill to medium. Grill the kebabs for 12–15 minutes, turning once and brushing with the remaining marinade.

Serve with a green or rice salad.

# *Mackerel Stuffed with Spinach*
### SERVES 4

1 small onion, peeled and finely chopped
3 slices bread, toasted and made into crumbs
115g (4oz) frozen spinach
4 small mackerel, gutted and heads removed
4 tablespoons lemon juice
salt and pepper to taste

*for the sauce*
2 tablespoons fresh chopped parsley
225g (8oz) low fat crème fraîche

Preheat the oven to 190°C, 375°F or Gas mark 5.

Dry-fry the onion for 5 minutes in a non-stick frying pan until soft (add a little water if it starts to burn). Add the breadcrumbs and cook until crisp. Remove from the heat and season well with salt and pepper. Add the spinach and stir well to mix.

Rinse the fish in cold water and pat dry with a kitchen towel. Open the cavity in each fish. Drizzle 2 tablespoons of the lemon juice in each cavity. Fill with the breadcrumb mixture and place in an oven-proof dish. Spoon the remaining lemon juice over each fish and bake in the oven for 20–25 minutes.

Mix the chopped parsley with the crème fraîche and serve with the fish.

Serve with a tomato salad.

# Mariner's Mediterranean Pie

## SERVES 4

1 fish or vegetable stock cube
350g (12oz) cod fillets, skinned
1 small can chopped tomatoes, drained
1 onion, peeled and chopped
½ red pepper, deseeded and chopped
½ green pepper, deseeded and chopped
1 teaspoon chopped mixed herbs
salt and pepper to taste
2 medium-sized potatoes, very thinly sliced

Preheat the oven to 180°C, 350°F or Gas mark 4.

Dissolve the stock cube in a little boiling water in a shallow pan. Add the fish and gently poach until soft (approximately 6 minutes). Drain and flake into a large ovenproof pie dish.

Stir in the drained tomatoes, onion, peppers, herbs and seasoning. Layer the potato slices on top so that they overlap each other until the whole of the pie is covered. Cover with foil and bake in the centre of the oven for about 1 hour.

Remove the foil and brown under the grill before serving.

# *Stuffed Plaice*

### SERVES 4

4 small plaice fillets, skinned
115g (4oz) prawns, shelled and cooked
150ml (¼ pint) white wine
1 packet white sauce mix
300ml (½ pint) skimmed or semi-skimmed milk in
addition to allowance
salt and pepper to taste
chopped parsley

Preheat the oven to 180°C, 350°F or Gas mark 4.

Place the prawns on the plaice fillets from the pointed end to halfway up. Roll up the plaice from the pointed end and place in an ovenproof dish. Pour the wine over. Cover with foil and cook in the oven for 20 minutes.

Make up the sauce according to the instructions on the packet, using the skimmed or semi-skimmed milk. Season with salt and pepper and pour over the fish. Sprinkle the chopped parsley over.

Serve with new potatoes and fresh green vegetables.

# Creamy Tuna Pasta

### SERVES 4

1 medium-sized onion, peeled and finely chopped
3–4 sticks celery, finely chopped
1 clove garlic, peeled and crushed (optional)
1 × 400g (14oz) can chopped tomatoes
1 × 185g (6½oz) can tuna in brine, drained
115g (4oz) mushrooms, thinly sliced
1 small tin sweetcorn, drained
salt and pepper to taste
1 standard tub of Shape plain soft cheese

In a large non-stick pan cook the onion, celery and garlic (if used) in the tomatoes until reasonably soft (approximately 5 minutes).

Add the tuna, mushrooms, sweetcorn and seasoning. Cook for approximately 5 more minutes.

Add the cheese and stir until it melts into the other ingredients.

Serve with pasta (50g/2oz uncooked weight per person), or jacket potatoes, and green salad, or on French bread (50g/2oz per person) as a pizza-style dinner.

# *Tuna Fish Pasta*

### SERVES 2

1 × 400g (14oz) can chopped tomatoes
1 tablespoon tomato purée
1 clove garlic, peeled and crushed
1 teaspoon dried basil
200g (7oz) pasta shapes
1 × 185g (6½oz) can tuna in brine, drained

Place the tomatoes, tomato purée, garlic and basil in a saucepan. Bring to the boil and simmer for approximately 15–20 minutes until the liquid has reduced and thickened.

Meanwhile cook the pasta in boiling salted water for 8 minutes. When cooked, drain and place in a serving bowl.

Add the tuna to the tomato sauce. Warm through, and then add to the pasta.

Serve immediately.

# *Tuna Rice Bake*

### SERVES 2

115g (4oz) long-grain rice
115g (4oz) frozen sweetcorn
1 medium onion, peeled and chopped
1 medium green pepper, deseeded and chopped
200g (7oz) mushrooms, chopped
1 teaspoon tomato purée
1 × 400g (14oz) can baked beans
1 × 185g (6½oz) can tuna in brine, drained
1 teaspoon mixed herbs

Cook the rice and sweetcorn in a pan of boiling salted water for 10 minutes.

Dry-fry the onion, green pepper and mushrooms in a non-stick pan with the lid on. When soft, add the tomato purée, beans, tuna and herbs and heat thoroughly.

Drain the rice and sweetcorn and place in a serving dish. Top with the sauce. Maintenance dieters may sprinkle 25g (1oz) grated low-fat Cheddar over.

## Tuna Rice and Peas

### SERVES 2

50g (2oz) (uncooked weight) long-grain rice
225g (8oz) frozen peas
1 × 185g (6½oz) can tuna in brine
4 teaspoons vinegar
4 teaspoons low-fat salad dressing
1 onion, peeled and finely chopped
50g (2oz) sultanas (optional)

Cook the rice and peas together in a pan of boiling water for 10 minutes.

Drain and flake the tuna. Mix together the vinegar and low-fat dressing. Drain the rice and peas and rinse with cold water.

Place all the ingredients, including the onion and sultanas (if used), in a salad bowl and gently mix together.

Serve cold with salad.

This dish can be kept refrigerated for a day or

two. It can be served with any salad and is also a marvellous packed lunch.

## *Tuna Sauce with Pasta*

SERVES 4

1 large onion, peeled and sliced
175g (6oz) mushrooms, wiped and sliced
1 vegetable stock cube
1 packet cheese sauce mix
300ml (½ pint) skimmed or semi-skimmed milk in
addition to allowance
1 × 185g (6½oz) can of tuna in brine
salt and pepper to taste

Cook the onion and mushrooms until soft in a small amount of water with the stock cube added.

Make up the cheese sauce as per packet instructions using the skimmed or semi-skimmed milk. Add the sauce to the onions and mushrooms. Drain and flake the tuna and add to the pan. Warm through and season with salt and pepper.

Serve over pasta of your choice (50g/2oz uncooked weight per person) or new or baked potatoes with a salad or vegetables.

# *Tuna and Tarragon Pasta*

### SERVES 1

50g (2oz) wholewheat pasta
1 × 185g (6½oz) can tuna in brine
1 tablespoon fresh tarragon
1 tablespoon tarragon vinegar (or cider vinegar
if not available)
1 tablespoon tomato ketchup
1 tomato, chopped
50g (2oz) canned peas
50g (2oz) canned sweetcorn
freshly ground black pepper

Cook pasta in boiling salted water for 8 minutes.

Drain and flake the tuna and mix with the tarragon, tarragon or cider vinegar and ketchup.

Place the tomato, peas, sweetcorn and tuna and tarragon mixture in a saucepan. Mix and heat thoroughly.

Drain the pasta and top with the sauce.

Serve with a generous grinding of freshly ground black pepper.

## MAIN COURSES:

## SIMPLE VEGETARIAN RECIPES

### *Bean Pie*

SERVES 1

1 small onion, peeled and sliced
225g (8oz) potatoes, peeled and sliced
115g (4oz) canned mixed beans
50g (2oz) mushrooms, sliced
1 small can tomatoes in juice
1 teaspoon soy sauce
$\frac{1}{2}$ teaspoon mixed dried herbs
salt and pepper to taste

Preheat the oven to 180°C, 350°F or Gas mark 4.

Cook the onion in a small basin in the microwave for 2 minutes until just soft. Arrange the potato slices in a thin layer on a plate and cook in the microwave for 4 minutes until just soft. Alternatively, cook the onion and potatoes in a saucepan with water until just soft.

Mix together the onion, beans, mushrooms, tomatoes, soy sauce and herbs. Season with salt and pepper. Place in a shallow ovenproof dish.

Arrange the potatoes on top of the bean mixture. Sprinkle with a little salt and bake in the oven for approximately 20–30 minutes until the potatoes are brown.

Serve with unlimited vegetables.

# *Bean and Vegetable Bake*

### SERVES 4

225g (8oz) carrots, diced
1 small cauliflower, chopped
675g (1½lb) potatoes, peeled and sliced
1 onion, peeled and sliced
450g (1lb) white cabbage, shredded
225g (8oz) mushrooms, trimmed
1 × 400g (14oz) can baked beans
1 × 400g (14oz) can chopped tomatoes
1 tablespoon mixed dried herbs
salt and black pepper to taste
1 tablespoon Parmesan cheese

Preheat the oven to 160°C, 325°F or Gas mark 3.

In one pan boil the carrots and cauliflower for 5 minutes. In another pan boil the potatoes for 15 minutes. In a third pan boil the onion and cabbage for 5 minutes. When cooked, drain the vegetables.

Place the carrots, half the mushrooms and all the beans into a large casserole or lasagne dish. Place the onion and shredded cabbage on top, followed by the chopped tomatoes, herbs, salt and plenty of black pepper. Cover with the cauliflower and sliced potato. Place the remaining mushrooms on top of the sliced potatoes. Sprinkle on the Parmesan cheese and more black pepper.

Bake in the oven for 30 minutes or until the vegetables are cooked.

Serve immediately.

# Broccoli Bake

## SERVES 4

500g (1¼lb) broccoli cut into florets
1 x 295g (11oz) can Campbell's Condensed Half Fat
Mushroom Soup
150ml (¼ pint) skimmed or semi-skimmed milk in
addition to allowance
115g (4oz) button mushrooms, sliced
150g (5oz) half-fat Cheddar cheese, grated
2 tablespoons fresh wholemeal breadcrumbs

Cook the broccoli in boiling water for 6–8 minutes or until tender. Drain.

Combine the soup, milk, mushrooms and half the grated cheese in a saucepan. Heat through gently until hot. Simmer for 2 minutes, stirring regularly.

Place the broccoli in a warmed 1.2 litre (2 pint) flame-proof dish and pour the sauce over. Sprinkle the remaining cheese and the breadcrumbs over the broccoli. Place under a preheated medium grill for 2–3 minutes or until golden brown.

# Cauliflower and Courgette Bake

### SERVES 4

2 onions, peeled and sliced
1 small to medium cauliflower, cut into florets
350g (12oz) courgettes, thickly sliced
1 egg
65g (2½oz) low-fat fromage frais or yogurt
2 teaspoons cornflour
½ teaspoon French mustard
salt and pepper to taste
115g (4oz) low-fat Cheddar cheese, diced
25–50g (1–2oz) wholemeal breadcrumbs
2–3 teaspoons Parmesan cheese (optional)

Preheat the oven to 190°C, 375°F or Gas mark 5.

Cook the onions in boiling salted water until they are almost tender. In a separate pan of boiling salted water, blanch the cauliflower florets for 5 minutes, then add the courgettes and cook for a further 2 minutes. Drain and rinse the onions, cauliflower and courgettes under cold running water until they are cold. Drain well again and place in an ovenproof dish.

Beat the egg well and mix with the fromage frais or yogurt, cornflour and mustard. Season with salt and pepper. Beat well until smooth. Add the Cheddar cheese and pour the mixture over the vegetables. Sprinkle the breadcrumbs and Parmesan cheese (if using) over the top.

Bake in the oven for about 25 minutes.

# Chickpea Couscous

### SERVES 4

1 tablespoon sunflower or vegetable oil
2 medium carrots, peeled and halved lengthwise and
sliced across
1 medium or large potato, peeled and chopped
½ cauliflower, cut into florets
225g (8oz) courgettes, chunkily chopped
50–75g (2–3oz) green beans, cut in half across
1 teaspoon ground coriander
2 vegetable stock cubes
450ml (¾ pint) water or light stock
150ml (¼ pint) ready-made tomato sauce
1 medium red pepper, deseeded and diced
115g (4oz) okra, topped and tailed and cut
in half across
2 green chillies
1 tablespoon tikka paste or other marinating paste
1 x 400g (14oz) can chickpeas, drained and rinsed
salt and freshly ground pepper

Heat the oil in a medium-sized saucepan and gently
fry the carrots, potato and cauliflower. Stir the mixture from time to time to prevent it sticking to the
bottom of the pan. Add the courgettes, green beans
and coriander and cook slowly for another 5
minutes.

Add the stock cubes, water or stock, tomato sauce,
red pepper, okra, chillies, tikka paste and chickpeas
and cook for 20–30 minutes.

Season well and serve hot on a bed of cooked

couscous, quinoa or rice (50g/2oz uncooked weight per person).

## Flat Stomach Plan Pizza

SERVES 2

*for the base*
300g (11oz) strong plain white or mixed wholemeal and white flour
1 rounded teaspoon easy-to-blend dried yeast
1 level teaspoon salt
150ml (¼ pint) warm water

*for the topping*
6 onions, peeled and sliced
2 cloves garlic, peeled and crushed
120ml (4fl oz) water
½ chicken stock cube
tomato paste or relish

Preheat the oven to 200°C, 400°F or Gas mark 6.

Place the flour, yeast and salt in a mixing bowl and, using a wooden spoon, mix to a soft dough.

Turn out on to a floured board and knead well for 5 minutes. Divide the dough into 2 pieces. Roll each out to form 2 × 23cm (9in) rounds and leave to rise slightly.

To make the topping, place the onions and garlic with the water in a frying pan. Cook gently over a low heat for approximately 20 minutes until very soft (slow cooking is important to get the right consistency). Add the stock cube and stir to dissolve. Add a little more water if needed.

Spread the tomato paste or relish on the pizza bases and spread the onion topping over. Place the pizzas in 2 × 23cm (9in) pizza pans. Bake in the oven for 15 minutes until the base is cooked.

## Hearty Hotpot

### SERVES 4

1 onion, peeled and chopped
450ml (¾ pint) vegetable stock
175g (6oz) carrots, chopped
2 bay leaves
1 teaspoon caraway seeds
115g (4oz) parsnips, peeled and chopped
115g (4oz) swede, peeled and chopped
350g (12oz) potatoes, peeled and diced
175g (6oz) Brussels sprouts, halved
115g (4oz) canned blackeye beans,
drained and rinsed
4 tomatoes, chopped
3 tablespoons red wine
2 teaspoons soy sauce
salt and black pepper

Dry-fry the onion in a non-stick saucepan until soft.

Add 120ml (4fl oz) vegetable stock, the carrots, bay leaves and caraway seeds and stir for a few minutes. Then add the parsnips, swede and potatoes and cook for a further 3–4 minutes. Add the

Brussels sprouts, beans, tomatoes, the remainder of the stock, the red wine and soy sauce; stir well and season to taste. Cover and cook for a further 30 minutes.

Remove the bay leaves and serve.

## Saucy Vegetables and Pasta
### SERVES 1

75g (3oz) pasta shells
1 onion, peeled and chopped
1 courgette, chopped
50g (2oz) mushrooms, chopped
1 teaspoon Worcester sauce
salt and pepper to taste
1 small can chopped tomatoes
1 level teaspoon sugar

Cook the pasta shells for 8 minutes in a pan of boiling salted water.

Cook the onion and courgette together in a saucepan in a little water until soft. Add the mushrooms, Worcester sauce, salt and pepper, tomatoes and sugar and cook for a further 5 minutes.

Drain the pasta shells. Mix the sauce into the pasta and serve.

# Soya Mince and Potato Pie

### SERVES 2

1 packet original Beanfeast soya mince
8 button mushrooms, sliced
½ cup frozen peas
½ onion, peeled and finely chopped
1 clove garlic, peeled and crushed
2 large potatoes
1 tablespoon skimmed or semi-skimmed milk in
addition to allowance
salt and pepper to taste

Preheat the oven to 190°C, 375°F or Gas mark 5.

Mix the Beanfeast according to the packet instructions, adding the mushrooms, peas, onion and garlic. Bring to the boil and simmer as directed.

Place the potatoes in a saucepan with water. Bring to the boil and cook until soft. Drain and mash with the milk and season with salt and pepper.

When the Beanfeast is cooked, place it in a small casserole dish. Place the mashed potatoes on top and smooth over with a fork.

Bake in the oven for 20 minutes or until the potatoes are browned.

Serve with unlimited vegetables.

# Spinach and Pasta Bake

### SERVES 4

1 x 400g (14oz) pack frozen spinach
2 onions, peeled and sliced
2 cloves garlic, peeled and crushed
400g (14oz) mushrooms, sliced
1 x 295g (11oz) can Campbell's Condensed Soup
(asparagus or mushroom)
skimmed or semi-skimmed milk in
addition to allowance
300g (11oz) 'no pre-cook' lasagne
450g (16oz) low-fat cottage cheese

Preheat the oven to 190°C, 375°F or Gas mark 5.

Cook the spinach according to the packet instructions. Drain and squeeze out all excess water.

Dry-fry the onion and garlic in a non-stick frying pan. Add the mushrooms to the pan with 2 tablespoons of water. Cover and heat quickly until nearly cooked.

Heat the soup in a saucepan, adding an equal amount of milk.

In a large ovenproof dish, place a layer of pasta and then alternate layers of the mushroom and onion mixture, spinach, cottage cheese then soup. Repeat until all the ingredients are used up, finishing with a layer of soup. Bake in the oven for about half an hour until bubbling.

Serve with a green salad or crusty soda bread 50g (2oz) per person.

# Stuffed Marrow

### SERVES 4

2 medium onions, peeled and finely chopped
2 cloves garlic, peeled and crushed
2 slices granary bread made into breadcrumbs
salt and freshly ground pepper to taste
2 teaspoons each dried chives and parsley
1 packet white sauce mix
300ml (½ pint) skimmed or semi-skimmed milk in
addition to allowance
1 bunch broccoli, cut into small florets
2 medium-sized marrows, peeled and deseeded

*to garnish*
sprinkling of chopped fresh coriander

Preheat the oven to 180°C, 350°F or Gas mark 4.

Dry-fry the onions and garlic in a non-stick pan until soft but not brown. Place in a large bowl. Add the breadcrumbs, seasoning and herbs to the bowl and mix together.

Make up the white sauce mix using all the milk. Pour into the bowl and mix thoroughly until the dry ingredients are coated with the sauce.

Steam or microwave the broccoli florets until just soft. Add to the mixture in the bowl.

Cut each marrow in half. Lay each half on a piece of foil approximately 38cm (15in) square. Fill the marrow halves with the mixture in the bowl.

Seal the foil around each marrow to make two parcels. Place on an ovenproof tray and bake for 25 minutes.

Remove the tray from the oven and undo the foil parcels. Pour away the excess juice, leave the marrows unsealed and replace in the oven for a further 5 minutes. Serve immediately with jacket potatoes garnished with coriander, plus vegetables of your choice.

# Vegetable Croquettes

### SERVES 1

115g (4oz) mashed potatoes
50g (2oz) sage and onion stuffing mix
115g (4oz) any frozen mixed vegetables
1 small onion, peeled and grated
salt and pepper
1 egg, beaten
breadcrumbs to coat

Preheat the oven to 180°C, 350°F or Gas mark 4.

Bind all the ingredients together with half of the beaten egg.

Shape the mixture into croquettes. Dip the croquettes in the remaining egg and roll in the breadcrumbs. Place the croquettes on a baking tray and bake in the oven for approximately 15 minutes or until golden brown.

Serve with Parsley Sauce (see recipe, page 246).

# *Veggie Delight*

SERVES 4

1 green pepper, deseeded and sliced
1 red pepper, deseeded and sliced
1 yellow pepper, deseeded and sliced
2 courgettes, sliced
1 onion, peeled and sliced
115g (4oz) mushrooms, sliced
1 small can tomatoes
2 tablespoons fresh oregano or basil
1 jar pasta sauce (e.g. Dolmio)
salt and pepper
1 cup water

Place all the ingredients in a saucepan. Bring to the boil, cover and simmer for 30 minutes or until the vegetables are soft.

Serve with pasta (50g/2oz uncooked weight per person) or jacket potatoes.

# Wyn's Wonderful Pasta

### SERVES 4

1 green, yellow or red pepper, deseeded and chopped
1 onion, peeled and chopped
1 carrot, peeled and chopped
1 or 2 cloves garlic, peeled and crushed
6 mushroom stalks, chopped (reserve the bodies and slice them)
1 green chilli, chopped (optional)
bunch of fresh basil
1 × 400g (14oz) can plum tomatoes
salt and pepper
225g (8oz) pasta shapes

Place all the ingredients except the pasta and reserved mushroom slices in a food processor and whizz until smooth to form a sauce.

Boil the pasta in a saucepan with water for approximately 8 minutes. Drain.

Place the sauce in a saucepan, add the sliced mushrooms and heat.

Stir in the pasta, heat through and serve immediately.

## MAIN COURSES:

### GOURMET MEAT RECIPES

# *Barbecued Pork Pouches*

SERVES 4

1 small onion, peeled and finely chopped
1 clove fresh garlic, peeled and crushed or
$\frac{1}{2}$ teaspoon garlic paste
50–75g (2–3oz) mushrooms, trimmed and finely
chopped
1–2 teaspoons curry powder
3 tablespoons tomato purée
salt and pepper to taste
2 tablespoons fresh breadcrumbs
4 × 175g (4 × 6oz) lean loin pork chops
$\frac{1}{2}$ teaspoon cinnamon
$\frac{1}{4}$ teaspoon ground cloves
good pinch of nutmeg
1 teaspoon brown sugar
300ml ($\frac{1}{2}$ pint) cider
1 teaspoon arrowroot

Dry-fry the onion and half the garlic in a frying pan
until they are almost soft.

Add the mushrooms to the pan and continue cooking until the mushrooms are soft and the mixture is
dry. Remove from the heat, then stir in the curry
powder and 1 tablespoon of the tomato purée.
Season well with salt and pepper, then stir in the
breadcrumbs.

Trim all the fat from the chops and make a deep

slit in the side of each right up to the bone to form a large pocket. Divide the mushroom and onion mixture into 4 and place a portion in each pocket. Press well in and press the edges together to seal in the mixture.

Mix the remainder of the garlic and tomato purée in a flat dish and stir in the cinnamon, ground cloves, nutmeg and brown sugar. Season lightly with salt and pepper and moisten with half the cider. Place the chops in the marinade and coat them well. Leave for 1–2 hours, turning occasionally.

Drain the marinade from each chop and reserve. Cook the chops over a preheated barbecue or under a preheated grill for 8–10 minutes on each side or until the meat looks cooked down the centre of the bone.

Meanwhile, mix the remainder of the marinade and cider together. Make this up to 300ml (½ pint) with water and place in a small pan and bring to the boil. Mix the arrowroot with a little cold water and add to the pan. Bring to the boil again, stirring all the time, and then check the seasoning. Serve with the cooked chops.

# Cassoulet

## SERVES 4

1 × 400g (14oz) can white haricot beans, drained
1 large onion, peeled and roughly chopped
450g (1lb) potatoes, peeled and cut into
even-sized pieces
500g (1¼lb) lean pork, cut into 2.5cm
(1in) cubes
1 × 400g (14oz) can chopped tomatoes
salt and freshly ground black pepper
1 teaspoon mustard powder
150ml (¼ pint) beef stock

Preheat the oven to 180°C, 350°F or Gas mark 4.

Mix together the beans, onion, potatoes, pork and tomatoes in a large casserole dish. Season well. Dissolve the mustard in the stock and pour over the casserole.

Cover and cook for 1½–2 hours until the pork is tender.

Serve with unlimited fresh green vegetables

# Beef and Mushroom Kebabs

## SERVES 4

400g (1lb) topside beef or rump steak
8 small onions, peeled
8 small mushrooms, washed and trimmed

Beat the beef well and cut into 16 thin slices. Wrap each onion and mushroom in a slice of beef.

Thread the beef rolls on to 4 skewers. Place under a hot grill for approximately 7–10 minutes.

Serve with salad.

## Beef Teriyaki Skewers

### SERVES 4

450g (1lb) rump steak, beaten and cut into 24 pieces
24 small new potatoes, scrubbed and cooked whole
8 spring onions, topped and tailed
2 large red peppers, deseeded and cut into squares
1 teaspoon Schwartz Onion Pepper
300g (12oz) (uncooked weight) brown rice
1 orange, cut into 8 segments

*for the marinade*
2 tablespoons dark soy sauce
2 tablespoons dry sherry
2 tablespoons soft brown sugar
2 tablespoons fresh ginger, peeled and finely grated
1 teaspoon Chinese five spice powder
1 clove garlic, peeled and crushed

Mix all the marinade ingredients together, add the steak and marinate overnight in a refrigerator.

On 8 skewers, alternate pieces of steak, potatoes, spring onions and red pepper. Sprinkle the skewers with the Onion Pepper and cook under a hot grill for 10–15 minutes until the steak is tender. Alternatively, barbecue until tender.

Meanwhile, boil the rice in salted water. Drain and rinse with cold water.

Place an orange segment on the end of each kebab and serve with a crisp green salad and the boiled rice.

## Chilli Con Carne

SERVES 4

450g (1lb) lean minced beef
1 large onion, peeled and chopped
1 × 400g (14oz) can chopped tomatoes
2 bay leaves
1 teaspoon Marmite or Bovril
1 × 425g (15oz) can red kidney beans, drained
1 teaspoon chilli powder (adjust according to individual taste)
2 cloves garlic, peeled and crushed
freshly ground black pepper

Dry-fry the mince in a non-stick pan. When cooked, drain through a sieve or colander and discard the fat.

Wipe away all the fat from the frying pan with kitchen paper, then add the onion to the pan and dry-fry. When the onion is just beginning to turn slightly brown, return the mince to the pan, add the tomatoes, bay leaves, Marmite or Bovril, kidney beans, chilli powder and garlic. Add liberal amounts of freshly ground black pepper. Heat through, adding water if the mixture becomes too thick.

Serve on a bed of boiled brown rice (50g/2oz uncooked weight per person).

# *Fillet of Beef with Peppercorns*

### SERVES 4

2 wine glasses white wine
1 tablespoon green peppercorns
4 × 175g (4 × 6oz) pieces of beef fillet
150g (5oz) low-fat natural yogurt
freshly ground black pepper to taste

Boil the wine with the peppercorns in a small saucepan until the liquid is reduced by half. Keep warm.

Heat the grill until it is really hot. Grill the beef fillets for 3 minutes on each side. Lower the grill pan and continue cooking until the fillets are cooked to your taste.

When the steaks are almost ready, bring the wine and peppercorn sauce back to boiling point. Remove from the heat and stir into it the natural yogurt, and season to taste. Return the pan to the heat for only a few seconds in order to heat the yogurt through. Do not allow it to boil or it will curdle.

Pour the yogurt, wine and peppercorn sauce over the steaks and serve with unlimited potatoes and other vegetables of your choice.

# *Hungarian Beef*

### SERVES 4

2 medium onions, peeled and chopped
4 tablespoons tomato juice
2 tablespoons paprika
675g (1½lb) stewing steak, cut into cubes
1 teaspoon caraway seeds
115g (4oz) potatoes, peeled and grated
2 tablespoons tomato purée
300ml (½ pint) stock
450g (1lb) potatoes, peeled and cubed
salt and freshly ground black pepper to taste

*to garnish*
1 green pepper, deseeded and sliced
fresh parsley, chopped

Preheat the oven to 180°C, 350°F or Gas mark 4.
Dry-fry the onions in a non-stick pan until brown.
Add the tomato juice and stir in the paprika. Add
the steak, caraway seeds and grated potato. Cook for
3–5 minutes, stirring occasionally.

Add the tomato purée and stock and transfer the
mixture to a casserole dish. Cover and cook for about
1½ hours. Add the cubed potatoes, season and cook
for a further 30 minutes. Check the seasoning.

Garnish with the pepper slices and parsley and
serve with a large green salad.

# Spicy Spaghetti Bolognese

## SERVES 4

450g (1lb) lean minced beef
1 large onion, peeled and chopped
1 × 400g (14oz) can chopped tomatoes
1 tablespoon tomato purée
2 tablespoons tomato ketchup or 120ml (4fl oz)
tomato juice
1 tablespoon brown sauce
$\frac{1}{2}$ teaspoon Tabasco sauce
2 level teaspoons chilli powder
2 cloves garlic, peeled and crushed, or $\frac{1}{2}$ teaspoon
dried garlic

Dry-fry the mince in a non-stick frying pan for 10 minutes, stirring frequently, until the meat changes colour. Drain the mince through a sieve or fine colander to remove all the fat.

Wipe out the frying pan with a piece of kitchen paper and dry-fry the onion until soft and brown. Return the mince to the frying pan. Add the chopped tomatoes and all the remaining ingredients. Mix well and cover. Cook on a low heat, stirring occasionally, for 45 minutes.

Serve with spaghetti (50g/2oz uncooked weight per person) and salad. Maintenance dieters may sprinkle a little Parmesan cheese over.

# Steak and Kidney Pie

## SERVES 4

225g (8oz) lean rump or sirloin steak, cut into cubes
225g (8oz) kidneys, cut into bite-sized pieces
2 medium-sized or 1 large onion, peeled
and chopped
300ml (½ pint) water
1 wine glass red wine
2 beef stock cubes
1 tablespoon gravy powder
900g (2lb) potatoes, peeled
2 tablespoons low-fat natural yogurt
4 tablespoons skimmed or semi-skimmed milk in
addition to allowance
salt and pepper to taste

Preheat the oven to 180°C, 350°F or Gas mark 4.

Heat a non-stick frying pan and dry-fry the cubes of beef steak and kidneys until well browned. Remove from the pan and place in a pie dish. Dry-fry the onion until soft and add this to the meat in the pie dish.

Place the water, wine and stock cubes in the pan and bring to the boil. Mix the gravy powder with a little cold water and add to the boiling stock in the pan, stirring continuously. The gravy should be quite thick. Add more gravy powder mixed with a little water as necessary. Pour the gravy over the meat in the pie dish.

Cook the potatoes in boiling salted water. Drain, then mash the potatoes with the yogurt and sufficient skimmed milk to make the consistency quite soft. Season to taste. Carefully spoon the potato on top of the meat and gravy to ensure that the meat is covered completely. Bake in the oven for 30–40 minutes, or until crisp and brown on top.

Serve with carrots and other vegetables of your choice.

## Kidney and Tomato Kebabs

### SERVES 4

4 lamb's kidneys
4 rashers lean bacon
1–2 green peppers
8 small tomatoes

Cut the kidneys in half, remove any membrane and the cores and soak in cold, lightly salted water for 30 minutes.

Stretch the bacon with a knife and cut each rasher in two. Roll up each rasher.

Remove the core, seeds and pith from the peppers and cut into 8 pieces.

Drain the kidneys well and thread all the ingredients alternately on to 4 skewers. Place under a hot grill for 5–7 minutes.

Serve with salad.

# Orange and Cranberry Kidneys

### SERVES 4

450g (1lb) lamb's kidneys, washed, cored
and quartered
1 medium onion, peeled and roughly chopped
175g (6oz) mushrooms, quartered
300ml (½ pint) beef stock
150ml (¼ pint) unsweetened orange juice
12.5g (½ oz) cornflour, blended with
2 tablespoons water
1 tablespoon fresh chopped parsley
1 tablespoon cranberry sauce
salt and freshly ground black pepper to taste

*for the border*
675g (1½lb) potatoes, peeled and diced
12.5g (½oz) very low-fat spread
1 tablespoon chopped fresh parsley or mint
thin strips of zest from ½ small orange, blanched in
boiling water

Boil the diced potatoes for 10–15 minutes until soft.
Drain and keep warm.

In a non-stick pan, dry-fry the kidneys and onion
for 2 minutes until the kidneys have browned. Add
the mushrooms and fry for a further 2 minutes.
Add the beef stock, orange juice and cornflour mixture. Bring to the boil, stirring continuously, and
cook for 10 minutes, stirring occasionally, allowing
the sauce to thicken and reduce. Add the parsley and
cranberry sauce and season well.

To make the border, add the low-fat spread, parsley

or mint and orange zest to the potatoes and toss until coated. Arrange as a border round the edges of a serving dish. Carefully spoon the kidneys into the centre of the dish.

Serve with green vegetables.

## *Lamb's Liver with Orange*

### SERVES 4

450g (1lb) lamb's liver
150ml (¼ pint) skimmed or semi-skimmed milk in addition to allowance
salt and freshly ground black pepper to taste
175ml (6fl oz) orange juice
¾ teaspoon arrowroot
¼ teaspoon chopped thyme

*to garnish*
1 orange, cut into slices

Remove any membrane or veins from the liver. Place in a bowl, pour the milk over and leave to stand for 1–2 hours if possible, but at least 30 minutes. This will keep the liver moist when it is cooked.

Dry-fry the liver in a non-stick pan until the liver is cooked but slightly pink in the centre, or cook under a preheated grill. When cooked, season with salt and pepper.

Heat the orange juice in a saucepan. Mix the arrowroot with a little water. Add to the pan and bring to the boil, stirring all the time.

Arrange the liver on a hot dish and pour the sauce

over. Sprinkle the thyme over the top. Garnish with
the orange slices just before serving.
Serve hot with vegetables.

# Liver with Red Wine and Rosemary

### SERVES 4

1 medium onion, peeled and finely chopped
1 clove garlic, peeled and crushed
450g (1lb) lamb's liver, thinly sliced
300ml ($\frac{1}{2}$ pint) beef stock
150ml ($\frac{1}{4}$ pint) red wine
1 teaspoon fresh chopped rosemary
175g (6oz) carrots, cut into julienne strips
2 teaspoons cornflour, blended with a little water
salt and freshly ground black pepper to taste

*for the border*
675g (1$\frac{1}{2}$lb) potatoes, peeled
1 teaspoon mixed dried herbs
salt and freshly ground black pepper

*to garnish*
fresh rosemary, chopped

Dry-fry the onion in a non-stick pan. Add the garlic
and continue cooking for approximately 2 minutes.
Add the liver and cook for 2 minutes, stirring continuously. Add the stock, wine, rosemary, carrots and
the blended cornflour. Bring to the boil, stirring all
the time. Season well. Cover the pan and simmer gently
for 45 minutes until liver and vegetables are tender.

Meanwhile, cook the potatoes in boiling water for approximately 15 minutes. Drain and mash. Mix the potato, herbs and seasoning together in a bowl. Transfer to a piping bag fitted with a large star nozzle and pipe a border around a shallow serving dish. Flash under a hot grill to brown.

Carefully spoon the liver into the centre of the dish. Garnish with rosemary and serve with green vegetables.

## MAIN COURSES:

## GOURMET CHICKEN RECIPES

# Chicken in Creamy Apple Sauce

### SERVES 4

4 chicken breasts, skinned
1 onion, peeled and finely sliced
1 clove garlic, peeled and crushed
150ml (¼ pint) apple sauce
150ml (¼ pint) chicken stock
150ml (¼ pint) cider
1 teaspoon dried tarragon
2 teaspoons cornflour, blended with a little water
salt and freshly ground black pepper to taste
150g (5oz) low-fat fromage frais

*for the border*
75g (3oz) low-fat fromage frais
675g (1½lb) potatoes, peeled, cooked and sieved

*to garnish*
fresh parsley, chopped

Preheat the oven to 180°C, 350°F or Gas mark 4.

Lightly dry-fry the chicken on both sides. Remove to a casserole dish. Dry-fry the onion and garlic for 2–3 minutes. Add the apple sauce, stock, cider, tarragon and blended cornflour. Stir continuously until the sauce comes to the boil. Season well. Pour the sauce over the chicken. Cover and cook in the oven for 1 hour.

When the chicken is almost ready, beat the fromage frais into the potatoes. Place in a piping bag fitted with a large star nozzle and pipe a double border of potato round a shallow serving dish. Flash under a hot grill to brown.

Remove the chicken from the oven, stir in the remaining fromage frais and arrange within the potato border. Garnish with parsley and serve with unlimited vegetables.

# Chicken and Mushroom Pilaff

### SERVES 4

225g (8oz) long-grain brown rice
900ml (1½ pints) chicken stock
6 spring onions, chopped
1 clove garlic, peeled and crushed
2 medium carrots, peeled and sliced
2 sticks celery, sliced
2 tablespoons water
2–3 teaspoons mild curry powder
2 teaspoons mango chutney
225g (8oz) cooked chicken, diced
225g (8oz) open cup mushrooms, wiped and halved
2 tablespoons fresh chopped coriander or parsley
salt and pepper to taste

*to serve*
8 tablespoons low-fat natural yogurt

Cook the rice in the chicken stock in a covered saucepan for 25–35 minutes, according to the instructions on the packet. The water should be absorbed but, if not, simmer it uncovered for an extra few minutes.

Place all the vegetables in a saucepan with the water, cover and simmer for 5 minutes. Add the curry powder and cook for 1 minute, then add the chutney, chicken and mushrooms and cook for 3 minutes. Stir in the rice, coriander or parsley, and seasoning. Cook until the rice is reheated.

Serve hot with spoonfuls of yogurt.

# Chicken and Mushroom Supreme

## SERVES 4

freshly ground black pepper
4 chicken breasts, skinned
soy sauce
225g (8oz) button mushrooms
2 teaspoons cornflour
6 tablespoons water

Preheat a non-stick frying pan and add a generous amount of freshly ground black pepper. Place the chicken in the hot pan and sprinkle more pepper on to the chicken. Sauté the chicken pieces until they have changed colour on all sides. Cover with a lid, reduce the heat and continue to cook on a low heat for 20–30 minutes. Add more pepper at approximately 10-minute intervals, at the same time turning the chicken over.

When the chicken is almost cooked add 6 tablespoons soy sauce to the frying pan. Add the button mushrooms, cover and simmer for a further 10 minutes. Add more soy sauce as necessary to prevent the pan becoming too dry.

When the chicken and mushrooms are thoroughly cooked, place them on a preheated serving dish and keep warm.

Add more soy sauce to the frying pan until there is approximately 150ml (¼ pint) fluid. Mix the cornflour and cold water together and carefully stir into the sauce in the pan. Remove from the heat as soon as it begins to thicken and stir vigorously to prevent it becoming lumpy. Return to the heat and cook gently for 2 or 3 minutes.

Serve with hot boiled rice (50g/2oz uncooked weight per person). Place the rice in a preheated serving dish and put the chicken pieces and mushrooms in the centre. Pour the hot sauce over the chicken and mushrooms and serve immediately, with unlimited green vegetables.

# Chicken à l'Orange

### SERVES 4

4 chicken breasts
1 wine glass red wine
3 oranges
1 large Spanish onion
onion salt and white pepper to taste
1–2 tablespoons redcurrant jelly
2 teaspoons cornflour
150ml (¼ pint) chicken stock

Remove any skin from the chicken breasts and leave to marinate in the red wine for 1 hour. Meanwhile squeeze the juice from the oranges and peel and slice the onion.

Preheat a non-stick frying pan and sprinkle with the onion salt and white pepper. When the pan is hot, add the chicken pieces (leaving the wine to one side for a moment), and sauté them on a brisk heat until they have changed colour, turning the chicken over to cook both sides. Add the onion or, if there is no room in the pan, dry-fry it in another non-stick frying pan. When the onion has become soft and brown add it to the chicken. Pour in the wine, orange juice and redcurrant jelly. Cover the pan and leave to simmer on a very low heat for 15 minutes or until the chicken is thoroughly cooked.

Meanwhile, mix the cornflour with the chicken stock. When the chicken is cooked, remove the chicken pieces from the pan and place on a pre-heated serving dish to keep warm. Gradually add the chicken stock and cornflour mixture to the pan and mix. Slowly bring to the boil, stirring all the time. Taste and adjust the seasoning if necessary.

When ready to serve, pour the orange sauce over the chicken pieces and serve immediately with unlimited potatoes and other vegetables.

## Chicken with Orange and Apricots

### SERVES 4

2 large oranges
1 onion, peeled and finely chopped
150ml (¼ pint) orange juice
150ml (¼ pint) dry white wine or cider
1 teaspoon arrowroot
4 chicken breasts or quarters
salt and pepper to taste
225g (8oz) fresh apricots or canned apricots in natural juice
1 tablespoon chopped fresh chervil or parsley

Preheat the oven to 180°C, 350°F or Gas mark 4.

Peel the rind from one orange very thinly and cut into fine (julienne) strips. Blanch in a little boiling water for 4–5 minutes until tender. Drain but reserve the water. Reserve the strips of peel for garnishing. Cut away the pith from this orange and then cut out the orange segments. Grate the rind from the other orange and squeeze out the juice.

Place the chopped onion in a pan with all the orange juice and the white wine or cider. Simmer gently until tender. Make the liquid up to 300ml ($\frac{1}{2}$ pint) with the reserved liquid. Mix the arrowroot with a little water and add to the pan. Bring to the boil, stirring all the time.

Skin the chicken and place in an ovenproof casserole. Pour the sauce over and season to taste with salt and pepper. Cover and cook in the oven for about 30–35 minutes until the chicken is almost tender.

Halve the fresh apricots and remove the stones, or drain the canned apricots. Add to the casserole and continue cooking for a further 10–20 minutes until the chicken and fruit are tender. Add the reserved orange segments about 5 minutes before the end of the cooking time so that they just heat through.

Check the seasoning. Pour into a hot dish or serve from the casserole. Sprinkle the strips of peel and the chervil or parsley over the top just before serving.

# Chicken in Orange and Marjoram

### SERVES 4

4 × 115g (4 × 4oz) chicken breasts, skinned
2 teaspoons dried marjoram
salt and freshly ground black pepper
2 medium oranges
1 teaspoon chicken seasoning
450g (1lb) potatoes, peeled, cut into matchsticks and
just cooked

*to garnish*
fresh chopped parsley

Preheat the oven to 200°C/400°F or Gas mark 6.

Open out the chicken breasts and sprinkle each with the marjoram. Season well. Cut one orange into 4 slices and halve each slice. Divide the pieces equally between the chicken and secure the meat around the orange with cocktail sticks. Squeeze the remaining orange and pour the juice into a shallow ovenproof dish. Add the chicken and sprinkle with the seasoning. Cover and cook for 20 minutes.

Place the potatoes around the edge to make a border and cook, uncovered, for a further 15 minutes or until the potato is golden. Garnish with parsley and serve with a crisp green salad and unlimited vegetables.

# Chicken with Paprika and Fennel

### SERVES 4

4 chicken joints, skinned and trimmed
1 teaspoon paprika
freshly ground black pepper
1 clove garlic, peeled and crushed
115g (4oz) lean smoked bacon, rinded and chopped
1 small leek, sliced
1 medium head fennel, chopped
115g (4oz) mushrooms, quartered
500g (1¼lb) new potatoes, scrubbed and cut into
even-sized pieces
1 tablespoon tomato purée
1 bouquet garni
600ml (1 pint) chicken stock
115g (4oz) green beans, topped and tailed
4 medium tomatoes, skinned and quartered
1 tablespoon cornflour, blended with a
little cold water

*to garnish*
fresh chopped parsley

Preheat the oven to 180°C, 350°F or Gas mark 4.

Sprinkle the chicken lightly with half the paprika and season with black pepper. Place the chicken, garlic and bacon in a large non-stick, flameproof casserole dish. Sauté for 5 minutes to seal the chicken. Remove from dish and set aside.

Dry-fry the leek, fennel and mushrooms for 3–4 minutes, adding a little warm stock if necessary. Stir in the remaining paprika, the potatoes, tomato purée and bouquet garni. Return the chicken to the casserole, pour over the stock and season well. Cover and cook in the oven for 40 minutes.

Remove the casserole from the oven and stir in the beans, tomatoes and blended cornflour. Return to the oven and cook for a further 20 minutes. Remove the bouquet garni. Garnish with parsley and serve with crusty bread (2oz/50g per person).

## Chicken Pilaff

### SERVES 4

1 large onion, peeled and finely chopped
1 green pepper, deseeded and finely chopped
600ml (1 pint) water
225g (8oz) long-grain rice
2 chicken stock cubes
350g (12oz) chicken
150ml (¼ pint) white wine
salt and pepper
115g (4oz) frozen peas
275–350g (10–12oz) canned sweetcorn

Cook the onion in a non-stick frying pan until soft and brown. Add the green pepper to the pan and continue dry-frying.

Meanwhile, bring the water to the boil in a large saucepan. Stir in the rice and the stock cubes. Continue cooking on a moderate heat until all the water has been absorbed and the rice is cooked. Stir frequently and add a little water as necessary to prevent sticking.

Skin, bone and chop the chicken into 1cm (½ inch) strips. Once the onion and pepper are cooked add the chicken and continue cooking. When the chicken has changed colour, add the wine and cook for a further 5 minutes. Sprinkle liberally with freshly ground black pepper, and salt if liked.

Lightly cook the peas and sweetcorn (these can be cooked together in one pan). Drain the peas and sweetcorn and add to the frying pan immediately. Stir the chicken-flavoured boiled rice into the chicken and vegetables. Serve straight away in a large preheated serving dish.

NB Do not rinse the rice after cooking as to do so would rinse away the chicken flavour.

## *Chicken and Potato Cakes*

### SERVES 4

350g (12oz) chicken meat, cooked
350g (12oz) potatoes, cooked
2 tablespoons skimmed or semi-skimmed milk in
addition to allowance (optional)
1 egg
2 tablespoons fresh parsley, finely chopped
1 teaspoon prepared mustard
salt and freshly ground black pepper to taste

Mince or very finely chop the cooked chicken. Mash the potatoes, adding the milk if they are too dry. Mix together the mashed potato and the chicken.

Add the egg, stir well, then add the parsley, mustard, salt and pepper. Wet your hands and form the chicken and potato mixture into small cakes.

Dry-fry in a non-stick frying pan until golden brown on each side.

Serve with unlimited vegetables.

## Chinese Chicken

### SERVES 1

175g (6oz) chicken, skinned and cut into strips
½ Spanish onion, peeled and coarsely chopped
1 teaspoon Schwartz Chinese seasoning
6 tablespoons water
2 tablespoons soy sauce
2 tablespoons lemon juice
115g (4oz) cut green beans
75g (3oz) cucumber, cut into 5cm (2in) lengths
½ red pepper, deseeded and cut into strips
115g (4oz) button mushrooms, cut in half
115g (4oz) beansprouts
75g (3oz) sweetcorn

Dry-fry the chicken and onion in a non-stick frying pan or wok for about 5 minutes. Stir in the Chinese seasoning, water, soy sauce and lemon juice. Bring to the boil. Reduce the heat and add all the other vegetables. Stir thoroughly and cook for approximately 5 minutes.

Serve piping hot on a plate with rice (50g/2oz uncooked weight per person).

# Glazed Chicken

### SERVES 4

4 chicken breasts, part-boned, or 8 chicken thighs
1 teaspoon French mustard
3 tablespoons tomato ketchup
1 tablespoon honey
1 tablespoon soy sauce
1 tablespoon lemon juice
¾ teaspoon ground ginger
2–3 drops Tabasco sauce or good pinch of cayenne pepper
300ml (½ pint) chicken stock
1 teaspoon arrowroot

*to garnish*
watercress
lemon wedges

Remove the skin from the chicken and make cuts in the flesh about 1cm (½in) apart. Place in a shallow dish.

Mix together the mustard, tomato ketchup, honey, soy sauce, lemon juice, ground ginger and Tabasco sauce or cayenne pepper. Spoon the mixture over the chicken pieces, cover and refrigerate for 3–4 hours. Spoon the marinade over the chicken occasionally.

Preheat the oven to 190°C, 375°F or Gas mark 5. Remove the chicken from the dish and place in a non-stick roasting tin. Reserve the rest of the marinade. Cook the chicken in the oven for 25–30 minutes until tender. Arrange on a hot serving dish.

Stir the stock into the remainder of the marinade

and mix well. Pour into a saucepan and bring to the boil. Mix the arrowroot with a little water and add to the pan. Bring to the boil again, stirring all the time.

Garnish the chicken with watercress and lemon wedges. Serve the sauce separately.

## Hot Chicken Surprise

SERVES 4

freshly ground black pepper
4 chicken breasts, all skin removed
225g (8oz) brown rice
450g (1lb) canned beansprouts
soy sauce

Preheat a non-stick frying pan and sprinkle generously with freshly ground black pepper. When the pan is hot, add the chicken pieces and sauté until they change colour and begin to brown. Sprinkle liberally with more black pepper and turn the chicken over to cook the other side. Reduce the heat, cover the pan with a lid and continue cooking for 20 minutes on a low heat, turning the chicken pieces over every 5 minutes or so. The steam trapped by covering the pan prevents the chicken from burning.

Meanwhile, cook the rice in boiling water and drain.

When ready to serve, drain the canned beansprouts and mix them together with the rice in a colander. Pour a kettle-full of boiling water over to reheat the rice and beansprouts. Drain well and place on a preheated serving dish. Top with the chicken pieces and serve with soy sauce to taste.

## MAIN COURSES:

## GOURMET FISH RECIPES

# Barbecued Fish Kebabs

### SERVES 4

500g (1¼lb) cod or halibut steak
2 servings Barbecue Sauce (see recipe page 245)
1 large onion, peeled and cut into medium-sized pieces
1 red pepper, deseeded and cut into squares
1 green pepper, deseeded and cut into squares
2 courgettes, thickly sliced
mushrooms, trimmed (optional)
12 cherry tomatoes (optional)

Cut the fish steaks into 2.5cm (1in) cubes and marinate in the barbecue sauce for at least 1 hour, preferably 2, before cooking.

Heat the grill and preheat 4 long or 8 short skewers if they are metal ones. Taking care not to burn your fingers, thread the vegetables and fish on to the hot skewers alternately until all the ingredients have been used up or the skewers are full. Brush the kebabs with the remaining barbecue sauce and place under a hot grill to cook, turning them frequently to prevent burning. Place any remaining vegetables on the grill pan to cook, and serve in addition to the kebabs.

When the kebabs are thoroughly cooked, serve them on a bed of boiled rice cooked in water with a fish stock cube. Heat any remaining barbecue sauce and serve separately.

## *Marinated Haddock*

### SERVES 4

350g (12oz) uncooked smoked haddock
1 medium onion, peeled and cut into rings
1–2 small carrots, cut into julienne sticks
1 teaspoon coriander seeds
2 bay leaves
2 lemons plus extra lemon juice if necessary
2 tablespoons white wine vinegar or cider vinegar
1 teaspoon caster sugar

*to garnish*
a few lettuce leaves
4 slices lemon (optional)
4 sprigs fresh parsley or chervil

Skin the haddock and remove any bones. Cut the fish into finger-sized 5cm x 1cm (2½in x ½in) strips and place in a shallow dish. Spread the vegetables and coriander seeds over the fish, and tuck the bay leaves under it.

Grate the zest from one lemon and squeeze the juice from both. Measure the juice and, if necessary, make up to 150ml (¼ pint) with extra juice. Mix the juice with the grated zest and vinegar, and pour over the fish. Sprinkle the caster sugar over the top. Cover and refrigerate for 8 hours or overnight.

To serve, arrange a few lettuce leaves on individual dishes. Remove the bay leaves and place some of the fish and vegetables in the centre of each dish. Pour over a little of the marinade. Garnish, if you wish, with a twist of lemon and a sprig of parsley or chervil. Refrigerate until you are ready to serve.

## *Prawn Pilaff*

### SERVES 4

450g (1lb) peeled prawns, fresh or frozen
600ml (1 pint) water
225g (8oz) long-grain rice
2 fish stock cubes
1 large onion, peeled and finely chopped
1 green pepper, deseeded and finely chopped
150ml (¼ pint) white wine
salt and pepper
115g (4oz) frozen peas
275–350g (10–12oz) canned sweetcorn

If you are using frozen prawns allow time for them to defrost completely. Rinse and drain the prawns, whether fresh or defrosted.

Bring the water to boil in a large saucepan and stir in the rice and the stock cubes. Continue cooking on a moderate heat until all the water has been absorbed and the rice is cooked. Stir frequently and add a little water as necessary to prevent sticking.

Meanwhile, dry-fry the onion in a non-stick frying pan until soft and brown. Add the green pepper and continue dry-frying until cooked. Add the wine and prawns and continue cooking for 5 minutes. Sprinkle liberally with salt and black pepper.

Lightly cook the peas and sweetcorn (these can be cooked together in one pan). Drain the peas and sweetcorn and add to the frying pan immediately. Stir the fish-flavoured boiled rice into the prawns and vegetables.

Serve immediately in a large preheated serving dish.

NB Do not rinse the rice after cooking as to do so would rinse away the fish stock flavour.

## Tagliatelle with Salmon and Scallops

### SERVES 4

350g (12oz) salmon tail fillet
lemon juice
freshly ground black pepper
150ml (¼ pint) medium white wine
175g (6oz) scallops
350g (12oz) tagliatelle (preferably verdi or spinach)
225g (8oz) low-fat fromage frais
½ teaspoon garlic granules or 1 clove garlic, peeled and crushed
½ teaspoon English mustard

Place the salmon on a microwave-safe plate and sprinkle with lemon juice and black pepper. Cover the top of the salmon with kitchen paper and place in the microwave for 4½ minutes on full power.

Remove from the oven, take off the kitchen paper and peel the skin from the fillet. Break the fish into large pieces with a fork and leave to cool.

Place 2 tablespoons of the wine, 2 tablespoons of water and 1 tablespoon of lemon juice in a non-stick pan and bring to the boil. Add the scallops and cover. Leave to boil for 1 minute, stirring occasionally to ensure the scallops do not stick. Remove from the heat and leave to cool.

Cook the tagliatelle in a large pan of boiling salted water for approximately 4 minutes, or according to the packet instructions.

Combine the fromage frais, garlic, mustard and the remaining wine in a bowl and mix until smooth. Add the drained scallops and salmon and combine together.

Drain the pasta, put into a large bowl with the sauce and fish and mix. Add more lemon juice and pepper to taste. Serve immediately.

## Trout with Herbs

### SERVES 1

1 trout
1 sprig each of parsley, dill, tarragon, sage and thyme
ground black pepper

*to garnish*
lemon wedges

Preheat the oven to 190°C, 375°F or Gas mark 5.
Remove the head and tail from the trout. Trim the

fins. Remove the gut and wash the fish well in cold water. Dry on kitchen paper.

Fill the cavity of the trout with herbs and black pepper. Wrap the trout loosely in two sheets of newspaper, and place under the tap to thoroughly wet the paper.

Place the trout, still wrapped in newspaper, on a non-stick baking tray. Bake in the middle of the oven for 30 minutes.

Remove from the oven. Slit open the newspaper and remove all the skin from the trout.

Garnish with lemon wedges and serve with unlimited vegetables.

## MAIN COURSES:

## GOURMET VEGETARIAN RECIPES

# Broccoli Gratiné with Cheese and Cannellini Topping

SERVES 4

*For the base*
450g (1lb) broccoli florets
175g (6oz) carrots, peeled and sliced

*for the topping*
1 × 400g (14oz) can cannellini beans,
drained and rinsed
175ml (6fl oz) semi-skimmed or skimmed milk in
addition to allowance
salt and freshly ground pepper
50–75g (2–3oz) low-fat Cheddar cheese, grated

*to garnish*
a few flaked almonds (optional)

Preheat the oven to 200°C, 400°F or Gas mark 6.

Steam the broccoli and carrots together until *al dente*.

Meanwhile, make the topping: blend the beans and milk together until smooth. Transfer the mixture to a saucepan, bring to the boil and simmer for 2–3 minutes. Season well and leave to cool.

Place the broccoli and carrots in a 1.5–1.75 litre (2½–3 pint) ovenproof dish. Pour the cannellini mixture over and top with the cheese. Sprinkle the almonds on top (if used).

Bake for 15 minutes or until golden.

Serve hot.

# Creamy Horseradish and Watercress Crumble

### SERVES 4

*for the base*
175g (6oz) cauliflower, cut into small florets
115g (4oz) broccoli florets
225g (8oz) courgettes, chopped
1 red pepper, deseeded and diced
50g (2oz) frozen garden peas
1 medium leek, peeled and chopped
25g (1oz) butter or margarine
25g (1oz) wholemeal plain flour
300ml (½ pint) skimmed or semi-skimmed milk in
addition to allowance
2 teaspoons creamed horseradish
½ bunch watercress, finely chopped
salt and freshly ground black pepper

*for the topping*
50g (2oz) wheat flakes, oat flakes or barley flakes
50g (2oz) wholemeal breadcrumbs
50g (2oz) butter or margarine
50g (2oz) low-fat Cheddar cheese, grated

*to garnish*
12.5g (½ oz) sunflower seeds

Preheat the oven to 190°C, 375°F or Gas mark 5.
   Steam the cauliflower and broccoli florets for 3 minutes. Add the courgettes and steam for another 2 minutes. Add the red pepper and peas and steam for another 2 minutes. Add the leek and steam for another 2 minutes.

Meanwhile, make the sauce. Melt the butter or margarine in a small saucepan and stir in the flour; cook the roux for 2 minutes. Take the pan off the heat and gradually add the milk, stirring all the time. Put the pan back on the heat and bring to the boil, stirring all the time. Turn the heat down and simmer for 3 minutes, still stirring. Take the pan off the heat again and stir in the horseradish, watercress and seasoning. Finally, fold in the steamed vegetables carefully.

Place the mixture in a 1.75 litre (3 pint) ovenproof dish.

Mix the flakes and breadcrumbs together. Rub the butter or margarine into the mixture and add the grated cheese.

Cover the vegetable mixture with the crumble topping and bake in the oven for 25 minutes or until crisp and golden on top.

Serve hot with a crisp salad.

# Egg and Vegetable Sauté

## SERVES 4

2 teaspoons olive oil
1 tablespoon vegetable oil
4 eggs, beaten
1 medium onion, peeled and roughly chopped
1 clove garlic, peeled and chopped
500g (1¼lb) potatoes, peeled, coarsely grated, rinsed
and dried
1 medium red pepper
115g (4oz) mushrooms, halved
4 tomatoes
115g (4oz) baby sweetcorn, halved
115g (4oz) mangetout, topped and tailed
115g (4oz) broccoli, broken into small florets
1 tablespoon tomato purée
2 tablespoons tomato ketchup
3 tablespoons light soy sauce
freshly ground black pepper

*to garnish*
fresh parsley, chopped

Heat the oils in a large non-stick frying pan or wok, add the beaten eggs and cook as an omelette for 2 minutes. Remove to a plate.

Fry the onion and garlic together in the same pan for 1 minute. Add the potato and stir-fry for 5 minutes. Add the remaining vegetables and fry, stirring occasionally, for a further 15–20 minutes until the potato is just cooked.

Roughly chop the omelette and add to the

vegetable mixture. Stir in the tomato purée, ketchup and soy sauce and cook for a further 5 minutes. Season well. Garnish with fresh parsley and serve with green vegetables.

## Lentil Roast

### SERVES 4

350g (12oz) orange lentils
1 bay leaf
2–3 parsley stalks
1 sprig fresh thyme
2 large onions, peeled and chopped
1–2 cloves garlic, peeled and crushed or
$1/2$–1 teaspoon garlic paste
2–3 sticks celery, sliced
$1/2$ green pepper, deseeded and diced
$1/2$ red pepper, deseeded and diced
1 dessert apple, peeled, cored and diced
75g (3oz) plain, low-fat quark or yogurt
salt and pepper to taste

Preheat the oven to 180°C, 350°F or Gas mark 4.

Wash the lentils well, drain and place in a large pan. Cover with water. (Do not add salt at this stage.) Tie the bay leaf, parsley stalks and thyme together with string and add to the pan. Bring to the boil.

Add the onions, garlic and celery to the lentils and simmer until the lentils and vegetables are tender and the liquid has almost evaporated.

When the lentils are tender, remove the bunch of

herbs and continue cooking, stirring all the time until the mixture is quite dry. Stir in the peppers and apples together with the quark or yogurt. Mix well and season to taste.

Pile the mixture into an ovenproof dish and bake in the oven for about 1 hour until the top is springy like a sponge.

Serve with a selection of seasonal vegetables.

## *Stir-fried Vegetables with Ginger and Sesame Marinade*

### SERVES 4

1½ tablespoons sunflower oil
1 onion, peeled, cut in half and shredded
350g (12oz) mangetout, topped and tailed
1 large red pepper, deseeded and cut into strips
275g (10oz) mung beansprouts
1 medium Chinese cabbage, shredded

### *for the marinade*
3 tablespoons fresh ginger juice (made by grating unpeeled root ginger and squeezing out the juice)
3 teaspoons arrowroot
3 tablespoons tamari
1 teaspoon toasted sesame oil
5 tablespoons light stock or water

Heat the oil in a wok or frying pan and quickly fry the onion until soft. Add the mangetout and cook for about 1 minute, stirring all the time to stop them from going brown. Add the red pepper and cook for another 3 minutes. Add the beansprouts and Chinese cabbage and cook until both look tender, stirring from time to time.

Meanwhile make the marinade by mixing all the ingredients together thoroughly. Add the marinade to the vegetables and bring the mixture back to the boil. Cover with a lid, turn the heat down and cook for a further 3–4 minutes to finish cooking the vegetables.

Serve straight away on a bed of cooked rice (50g/ 2oz uncooked weight per person).

## Three-Layer Millet Bake

### SERVES 4

225g (8oz) millet
2 teaspoons bouillon powder or 1½ vegetable stock cubes
450ml (¾ pint) water

*for the base*
1 tablespoon olive oil
1 onion, peeled and finely chopped
275g (8oz) courgettes, chopped
2 cloves garlic, peeled and crushed
1 × 400g (14oz) can chopped tomatoes
1–2 tablespoons tomato purée
1 teaspoon fresh mixed herbs
2 tablespoons fresh chopped parsley
salt and freshly ground black pepper

*for the topping*
300ml (½ pint) low-fat natural yogurt
115g (4oz) low-fat Cheddar cheese, grated
a good pinch of ground cumin

Preheat the oven to 190°C, 375°F or Gas mark 5.

Place the millet and the bouillon powder or stock cubes in a medium-sized saucepan. Add the water, bring the mixture to the boil, cover with a lid and simmer for 20 minutes.

Meanwhile, make the tomato sauce. Heat the olive oil and fry the onion, courgettes and garlic on a medium heat until tender. Add the tomatoes and tomato purée and boil for 5 minutes. Add the herbs and season.

To make the topping, place the yogurt in a mixing bowl and add the grated cheese and cumin.

Place the tomato mixture in a 1.5–1.75 litre (2½–3 pint) ovenproof dish, cover with the cooked millet and finish with the yogurt layer. Bake in the oven for 30 minutes or until the yogurt is set.

Leave to stand for 5 minutes and serve hot with a salad.

# Tikka Lentil Bake

### SERVES 4

*for the base*
175g (6oz) brown lentils
1 tablespoon sunflower or vegetable oil
175g (6oz) leeks, washed and chopped
2 cloves garlic, peeled and crushed
1 medium carrot, peeled and diced
115g (4oz) turnip, peeled and diced
225g (8oz) mushrooms, diced
2 tablespoons tomato purée
1 teaspoon Marmite dissolved in 2–3 tablespoons
boiling water
1 tablespoon tikka paste
2 tablespoons tamari (or other good quality soy
sauce)
salt and freshly ground black pepper

*for the topping*
450g (1lb) potatoes, peeled and chopped
12.5g (½oz) butter or margarine (optional)
4–6 tablespoons semi-skimmed or skimmed milk in
addition to allowance

Preheat the oven to 200°C, 400°F or Gas mark 6.

Bring 600ml (1 pint) water to the boil in a sauce-pan. Add the lentils and boil fast for 10 minutes uncovered. Turn the heat down and simmer for approximately 30 minutes until tender.

Meanwhile, heat the oil in a medium saucepan and fry the leeks until soft. Add the garlic, carrot, turnip and mushrooms, and cook, covered, for 10 minutes.

Make the topping by placing the potatoes in a saucepan with water and bringing to the boil. Simmer until tender, then drain and mash with a little butter or margarine and milk.

When the leeks and other vegetables are tender, add the cooked lentils, tomato purée, Marmite stock, tikka paste, tamari or soy sauce and salt and pepper. Bring the mixture to the boil and cook together for a few minutes for the flavours to mingle.

Place the lentil mixture in a 1.5–1.75 litre (2½–3 pint) oval ovenproof dish. Top with the mashed potatoes and finish with a decorative pattern, using a fork. You may sprinkle a few sesame seeds on the top and finish with a dot of butter to help with browning. Bake in the oven for 25 minutes.

Serve hot with a selection of steamed vegetables.

# Tricolour Pasta Risotto

### SERVES 4

1 tablespoon olive oil
1 onion, peeled, cut in half and shredded
225g (8oz) courgettes, thinly cut lengthwise – discard
the first slice, then cut into 4cm (1½in) long
pieces across
1 red pepper, cut into 4cm (1½in) long strips
75g (3oz) petits pois
225g (8oz) tricolour pasta spirals
450ml (¾ pint) water
1 vegetable stock cube
1 × 400g (14oz) can tomatoes
2 teaspoons freshly chopped or 1 teaspoon dry
marjoram
salt and freshly ground black pepper to taste
50g (2oz) strong low-fat cheese, grated

Heat the oil in a frying pan and fry the onion and courgettes for 3 minutes. Add the red pepper, peas, pasta, water, stock cube, tomatoes and marjoram. Bring to the boil, cover, and simmer for 20 minutes.

Season with the salt and pepper, then leave the mixture to stand for 5 minutes before serving.

Sprinkle with the cheese and serve with a crisp salad.

# *Vegetable Pilaff*

### SERVES 4

900ml (1½ pints) water
2 vegetable stock cubes
275g (10oz) brown rice
115g (4oz) frozen sweetcorn
115g (4oz) frozen peas
1 large onion, peeled and finely chopped
1 red pepper, deseeded and finely chopped
1 wine glass white wine
115g (4oz) canned red kidney beans, drained

In a large saucepan bring 600ml (1 pint) of the water to the boil, add the stock cubes and the brown rice. Bring back to the boil and simmer until the rice is soft but not overcooked. If the rice becomes too dry during cooking, add more water. If all the stock has not been absorbed at the end of cooking, drain the rice through a colander. However, do not rinse the cooked rice as this will remove the vegetable flavouring from the stock cubes.

In a small saucepan add the sweetcorn and peas to 300ml (½ pint) water. Bring to the boil, remove from the heat and drain.

Preheat a non-stick frying pan and cook the onion until it begins to turn brown. Then add the chopped pepper and cook until both are soft. Add the white wine, beans, peas and sweetcorn. Simmer on a very low heat until the wine has been reduced and absorbed by the vegetables. Keep it warm.

Add the cooked rice to the vegetables in the frying

pan and mix well. Serve immediately on a preheated serving plate.

## VEGETABLE ACCOMPANIMENTS

### Dry-roast Parsnips

SERVES 4

4–6 medium sized parsnips
salt

Preheat the oven to 200°C, 400°F or Gas mark 6.

Peel the parsnips and cut in half lengthways. Blanch by putting into cold salted water and bringing to the boil.

Drain thoroughly and sprinkle lightly with salt. Place on a non-stick baking tray without fat in the oven for about 30 minutes or until the parsnips are soft in the centre when pierced with a fork.

### Dry-roast Potatoes

SERVES 3

450g (1lb) medium-sized potatoes
salt

Preheat the oven to 200°C, 400°F or Gas mark 6.

Peel the potatoes, then blanch them by plunging them into cold water in a saucepan, together with a stock cube, and bringing to the boil.

Drain thoroughly. Lightly scratch the surface of each potato with a fork, and sprinkle lightly with salt.

Place on a non-stick baking tray, without fat, in the oven for about 1 hour.

## Lyonnaise Potatoes

SERVES 2–4

450g (1lb) potatoes, scrubbed and sliced
2 large Spanish onions, peeled and sliced
garlic granules
150–300ml ($\frac{1}{4}$–$\frac{1}{2}$ pint) skimmed or semi-skimmed
milk from allowance

*to garnish*
chopped parsley

Preheat the oven to 200°C, 400°F or Gas mark 6.

Place the potatoes and onion in layers in a casserole dish, sprinkling a few garlic granules between each layer. Pour over enough skimmed milk to almost reach the top layer of the vegetables. Cover and cook in the oven for 45 minutes to 1 hour until tender.

Garnish with chopped parsley and serve hot.

## Fat-free French Fries

SERVES 4

4 large baking potatoes (about 900g/2lb total weight)
2 egg whites
1 tablespoon Cajun spice

Preheat the oven to 200°C, 400°F or Gas mark 6. Place a non-stick baking tray in the oven to heat.

Slice the potatoes lengthwise into 5mm (4in) strips, then slice really thin into matchstick-shaped chips.

Gently whisk the egg whites with the Cajun spice until the egg whites are broken down and frothy. Slowly stir the potato sticks in the mixture until thoroughly coated.

Carefully place the potato sticks evenly on a pre-heated non-stick baking tray, keeping them in a single layer.

Place the baking tray in the centre of the oven and bake for 40 minutes or until the chips are crisp and brown, turning them every 10 minutes to enable even browning.

Serve immediately.

## Oven Chips

### SERVES 4

2–3 large potatoes
1 teaspoon oil

Preheat the oven to 220°C, 425°F or Gas mark 7.

Peel the potatoes and cut into chips. Blanch in boiling salted water in a saucepan for 5 minutes, then drain.

Meanwhile, brush a baking tray with the oil and place in the oven for 7–10 minutes until the oil is very hot.

Spread the chips over the baking tray and turn them gently so that they are lightly coated with the oil.

Bake on the top shelf of the oven for about 35–40 minutes (depending on the size of the chips) until they are soft in the middle and crisp on the outside. Turn the chips once or twice during the cooking time.

## *Potato and Onion Bake*

SERVES 4-6

450–675g (1–1½lb) old potatoes
175–225g (6–8oz) onions
300ml (½ pint) vegetable or chicken stock
salt and freshly ground black pepper

Preheat the oven to 220°C, 425°F or Gas mark 7.

Peel and thinly slice the potatoes and onions (the slicing attachment on a food processor or mixer is ideal for this purpose).

Place the stock in a saucepan and bring to the boil. Add the onions and cook for 3–4 minutes.

Place a layer of potatoes in the base of an oven-proof dish. Using a slotted spoon remove the onions from the stock and place them on top of the potatoes. Cover with the remainder of the potatoes. Season each layer lightly.

Pour the remaining stock over the potatoes, cover with a lid or foil and bake in the oven for 1–1¼ hours until the vegetables are tender. Check them once or twice while they are cooking and press them down so that the top layer is kept moist. Take off the lid for the last 20 minutes of the cooking time so that the potatoes turn golden brown on top.

## *Spicy Potatoes*

### SERVES 4

500g (1¼lb) potatoes, scrubbed
1 onion, peeled and finely sliced
300ml (½ pint) water
1 tablespoon soy sauce
2 teaspoons curry powder (optional)
1 teaspoon Worcester sauce

Cut the potatoes into small pieces. Place in a saucepan with the onion and water. Bring to the boil and cook until soft.

Drain the potatoes and onions. Return them to the pan and add the soy sauce, Worcester sauce and curry powder (if used).

Cook for a few minutes, stirring continuously to prevent sticking.

# Lemon-glazed Vegetables

## SERVES 4

450g (1lb) small new potatoes
175g (6oz) small new carrots
175g (6oz) French beans
175g (6oz) baby courgettes
115g (4oz) mangetout
115g (4oz) baby sweetcorn
65g (2½oz) sugar
2 teaspoons French mustard
4–5 tablespoons lemon juice
grated rind of 1 lemon
1 tablespoon chopped coriander

Scrape the potatoes and carrots, top and tail the French beans, courgettes and mangetout.

Cut each bean into 2–3 pieces. If the courgettes are very small just cut into 4 lengthways, otherwise cut in half and then quarter them lengthways.

Cook the potatoes in a pan of boiling salted water until tender.

In another pan of boiling salted water cook the carrots for about 4 minutes, then add the French beans and cook for a further 4–5 minutes. Finally, add the courgettes, mangetout and baby sweetcorn for a few minutes. Try and keep the vegetables slightly crisp.

Reserve about 150ml (¼ pint) of the vegetable water and drain the rest of the vegetables. Keep hot.

Add the sugar, mustard and lemon juice to the reserved vegetable water and boil until syrupy.

Return the vegetables to the pan and turn carefully to coat them with the glaze. Pile into a hot serving dish and sprinkle with the grated lemon rind and the chopped coriander just before serving.

# Spinach Roulade with Mushroom Filling

### SERVES 4

450g (1lb) frozen chopped spinach
4 egg whites
salt and pepper to taste
sprinkling of Parmesan cheese (optional)

*for the filling*
1 chicken stock cube
1 large onion, peeled and diced
2 garlic cloves, peeled and crushed
225g (8oz) mushrooms, sliced
$\frac{1}{2}$ teaspoon nutmeg
1 teaspoon chopped parsley
salt and pepper
1 tablespoon flour
50ml ($\frac{1}{4}$ pint) skimmed or semi-skimmed milk in addition to allowance

Preheat the oven to 220°C, 425°F or Gas mark 7.

Grease and line a Swiss roll tin with greaseproof or non-stick parchment.

Mash the spinach thoroughly and cook in a saucepan with a tiny amount of water until just cooked. Drain and cool.

Beat the egg whites until stiff and fold into the spinach. Season with salt and pepper. Quickly pour the mixture into the lined Swiss roll tin and sprinkle with Parmesan (if used). Bake on the top shelf of the oven for 15 minutes.

To make the filling place the chicken stock cube in a saucepan with 2 tablespoons of water. Add the onion and garlic and cook until nearly soft.

Add the mushrooms, nutmeg, parsley, salt and pepper and cook until the mushrooms are tender.

Mix the flour with the milk and stir into the saucepan to thicken.

Remove the spinach mixture from the tin and tip on to a clean tea towel. Remove the paper and spread the mushroom filling on top. Smooth the mixture evenly. Carefully roll up the roulade like a Swiss roll and place in a serving dish. Place in the oven to keep warm until you are ready to serve. Slice before serving.

## DESSERTS

### Apple Jelly with Fromage Frais

SERVES 4

450g (1lb) cooking apples
artificial sweetener to taste (optional)
1 packet jelly
2 cups water
115g (4oz) low-fat fromage frais

Peel and thinly slice the apples and place in a saucepan with a little water and artificial sweetener if desired. Cover with a tightly fitting lid and cook gently until stewed. Leave to cool. Spoon the apple into individual dishes.

Make up the jelly with the 2 cups of water and pour it over the apple in the individual dishes. Leave to set.

When ready to serve, top with the fromage frais.

## Autumn Pudding

### SERVES 6–8

7–9 slices white or brown bread
450–900g (1–2lb) mixed autumn fruits
(apples, pears, blackberries)
4 teaspoons water
5–6 tablespoons Canderel

Cut the crusts off the bread and line the base and sides of a 1.2 litre (2 pint) pudding basin, reserving 2 slices.

Prepare the fruit: peel, core and slice the apples and pears, and hull the blackberries. Place the apples and pears in a saucepan with the water. Cover with a tight-fitting lid and cook over a very gentle heat until just soft but not mushy. Remove from the heat and leave to cool. Stir in the Canderel and the hulled blackberries.

Using a slotted draining spoon, transfer the prepared fruit into the bread-lined basin. Add the remaining slices of bread. Cover with a piece of greaseproof paper, then place a saucer on top. Weight the saucer to encourage the juices from the fruit to soak into the bread. Refrigerate the pudding and remaining sauce overnight.

To serve, invert the basin on to a plate and pour the sauce over the pudding.

## Cheese and Apricot Pears

### SERVES 4

4 ripe pears
lemon juice
225g (8oz) low-fat cottage cheese
4 tablespoons apricot jam or preserve

Peel the pears, cut in half lengthways and remove the core. Brush with the lemon juice to prevent discoloration. Fill with the cottage cheese mixed with apricot jam or preserve. Serve chilled.

## Fresh Fruit Salad

### SERVES 10

2 oranges
1 small bunch green seedless grapes
2 kiwi fruit
3 red apples
2 pears
2 bananas

*for the syrup*
pared rind and juice of 2 lemons
2 tablespoons sugar
250ml (8fl oz) water

Peel the orange and cut into segments. Wash the grapes and peel the kiwi fruit. Core and slice the apples, leaving the skin on. Peel and core the pears.

To make the syrup, simmer the pared rind from the lemon in a saucepan with the water and sugar for approximately 5 minutes. Cool and strain. Add the lemon juice and pour over the fruit.

Put the fruit salad in the fridge until required. Just before serving, slice the banana and add to the salad.

# Fruit Crumble

### SERVES 4

450g (1lb) any soft fruit suitable for stewing
2 tablespoons water
2 tablespoons sugar
115g (4oz) fresh brown breadcrumbs (made from
4 slices bread)
50g (2oz) demerara sugar

Preheat the oven to 190°C, 375°F or Gas mark 5.

Place the fruit in a saucepan with the water and sugar. Cook on a gentle heat to stew the fruit until it is just soft.

Place the fruit in an ovenproof dish and cover with the breadcrumbs. Sprinkle the demerara sugar over and bake in the oven for 20 minutes.

Serve with low-fat custard or low-fat natural yogurt.

## *Fruit Delight*

### SERVES 4

450g (1lb) any soft fruit suitable for stewing
2 tablespoons sugar
2 tablespoons water
115g (4oz) low-fat fromage frais
1 × 150g (5oz) carton low-fat natural yogurt

*to decorate*
demerara sugar

Place the fruit in a saucepan with the sugar and water and cook gently until soft. When soft, place the fruit in a bowl and leave to cool.

When the fruit is cool add the fromage frais and stir until well mixed. Add the yogurt and mix thoroughly.

Pour the mixture into 4 individual dishes and sprinkle demerara sugar on top. Place in the refrigerator for an hour before serving.

## *Fruit Flan*

### SERVES 4–6

*for the flan case*
2 eggs
50g (2oz) caster sugar
½ teaspoon baking powder
50g (2oz) plain flour

*for the filling*
1 small can peaches in natural juice
glacé cherries
1 packet quick set gel

Preheat the oven to 200°C, 400°F or Gas mark 6.

Grease a 20cm (8in) sponge flan tin and sprinkle with flour.

Whisk the eggs and sugar together for 10 minutes until very thick and creamy.

Sift the baking powder and flour together and gently fold in the eggs. Pour immediately into the flan tin and bake on the middle shelf of the oven for 8–10 minutes.

Remove from the oven and allow to cool for a few minutes, then turn the flan case out on to a wire rack to cool completely.

When the flan case is cool, place it on a serving plate. Arrange the peaches and cherries in the cooled flan case. Make up the quick set gel according to the packet instructions. When the gel is cool enough, spoon it over the fruit. Place in the refrigerator until ready to serve.

## Ginger and Lemon Fluff

### SERVES 2

1 egg white
50g (2oz) caster sugar
1 small piece stem ginger, finely chopped
2 tablespoons freshly squeezed lemon juice
115g (4oz) oranges or mandarins

Whisk the egg white until it forms stiff peaks. Gradually whisk in the caster sugar. Whisk in the stem ginger and lemon juice. Place in the refrigerator until required.

This dish is best served within an hour of making. Serve with the oranges or mandarins.

# Home-made Ice Cream

### SERVES 4 – 6

1 × 410g (14½oz) can Lite Carnation Milk (chilled
overnight in fridge)
175g (6oz) granulated sugar
4 tablespoons water
1 sachet gelatine
2 teaspoons vanilla essence

Whisk the milk until thick and the volume has doubled.

Add the sugar and continue whisking.

Place the water in a small basin, sprinkle the gelatine on top and microwave on full power for 1 minute to dissolve. Allow to cool. When the gelatine has cooled pour it on to the milk and sugar mixture and continue to whisk. Mix in the vanilla essence, place in a container and freeze. Remove from the freezer 10 minutes before serving. The ice cream is best eaten within 48 hours.

## Variations

Any of the following flavourings can be used:

Coffee: whisk in 4 level tablespoons instant coffee powder.

Strawberry: whisk in the contents of a small can of strawberries and 1 teaspoon Supercook strawberry flavouring.

Rum and Raisin: whisk in 50g (2oz) raisins and 1 teaspoon Supercook rum flavouring.


# Kiwi and Ginger Dessert

### SERVES 4

1 ogen, or galia melon, halved and seeded
2 kiwi fruit, thinly sliced
225g (8oz) green grapes, halved and pitted
15g (½oz) stem ginger, thinly sliced
2 tablespoons ginger syrup (from the ginger)
4 tablespoons apple juice

Scrape the flesh from the melon with a melon-baller or cut into cubes. Place in a bowl with the kiwi fruit, grapes and stem ginger.

Mix the ginger syrup and apple juice together and pour over the fruit.

Serve in individual dishes.

# Low-fat Trifle

### SERVES 4

1 packet sugar-free jelly
2 medium-sized bananas, peeled and sliced
1 × 425g (17oz) carton low-fat custard
2 × 150g (5oz) vanilla virtually fat-free yogurt

In a large dish make up the jelly as instructed on the packet. Add the bananas and leave to set.

When set, cover the jelly with the low-fat custard, then smooth the yogurt over the top.

# Melon Sundae

### SERVES 4

450g (16oz) melon flesh
275g (10oz) low-fat yogurt, any flavour, or low-fat fromage frais
225g (8oz) green grapes

Finely chop the melon flesh and divide equally between 4 tall glasses. Spoon sufficient yogurt or fromage frais to cover the melon.

Wash, halve and seed the grapes. Divide them equally between the glasses (reserving 4 halves for decoration) placing them on top of the yogurt. Add the remaining yogurt or fromage frais and chill until ready to serve.

Before serving, place a grape half on top of each glass to decorate.

# Orange and Pineapple Jelly

## SERVES 2

120ml (4fl oz) water
1 packet gelatine
1 × 225g (8oz) can pineapple chunks in natural juice
120ml (4fl oz) orange juice

Place the water in a Pyrex measuring jug, sprinkle the gelatine on top and microwave on full power for 1 minute. Stir until the gelatine granules have dissolved.

Drain the liquid from the canned pineapple into the jug and top up with the orange juice to the 15fl oz (¾ pint) mark.

Place the pineapple pieces in a 600ml (1 pint) or 2 × 300ml (½ pint) bowls and pour the gelatine liquid over the fruit. Place in the refrigerator and leave to set.

Eat within 2 days.

# Peach Melba Jelly Dream

## SERVES 4

1 small can peach slices in natural juice
12 Boudoir biscuits or sponge fingers
1 packet sugar-free raspberry jelly
1 × 150g (5oz) very low-fat peach melba yogurt or virtually fat-free fromage frais

Drain the peaches and reserve the juice. Cut the peach slices in half and place in the bottom of a deep jelly mould. Arrange biscuits or sponge fingers vertically around the sides of the mould, cutting the excess off at the top.

Make up the jelly as directed on the packet, using the reserved peach juice and adding water to make up to a maximum of 450ml (¾ pint). Pour into the jelly mould over the peach slices, keeping the biscuits in place. Leave to cool in the fridge.

When the jelly is completely set, turn it upside down on to a plate and pour the yogurt or fromage frais over.

NB If you don't have a jelly mould, arrange the mixture in 3 layers, i.e. fruit, biscuit or sponge fingers, jelly.

## Pineapple Meringue

### SERVES 4

1 medium-sized can pineapple chunks or
crushed pineapple in natural juice
2 teaspoons cornflour
115g (4oz) sugar
2 trifle sponges
2 egg whites

Preheat the oven to 200°C, 400°F or Gas mark 6.

Drain the juice from the pineapple into a small saucepan and thicken with cornflour mixed with a little water. Add 25g (1oz) sugar.

Crumble the sponges into an ovenproof dish and arrange the pineapple chunks or crushed pineapple over the top. Pour the thickened juice over the top.

Whisk the egg whites until stiff, then whisk in the remaining sugar. Place over the pineapple mixture and bake in the oven for about 10 minutes until the meringue is set and browned.

## Pineapple Snow

### SERVES 4

1 medium-sized can crushed pineapple in
natural juice
1 packet sugar-free lemon jelly
1 × 150g (5oz) carton low-fat natural yogurt

Drain the pineapple and reserve the juice.

Make up the jelly according to the packet instructions using the reserved pineapple juice and water up to 600ml (1 pint). Add the crushed pineapple and leave to set.

When the jelly is set use a fork to break it up. Add the yogurt and mix in evenly using a fork.

## Strawberry Layer Dessert

### SERVES 4

1 packet sugar-free strawberry jelly
1 x 150g (5oz) carton low-fat natural yogurt
225g (8oz) fresh strawberries

Divide the jelly into 2 portions. Make up 1 portion using 100ml (3fl oz) water. Add the yogurt, mix well and pour into 1 large or 4 small dishes. Leave to set in the refrigerator.

Make up the remainder of the jelly using 200ml (7fl oz) water. Don't put it in the refrigerator. If it sets, melt it slightly again in the microwave.

When the yogurt jelly is set, arrange the strawberries on the top. Pour the remaining jelly over and leave to set.

## Strawberry Sorbet

### SERVES 4

450g (1lb) strawberries
2 large egg whites
liquid artificial sweetener to taste (optional)

*to serve*
additional fresh strawberries

Wash and hull the strawberries and place them in a large saucepan with very little water (just enough to prevent the strawberries sticking to the pan). Add a little artificial sweetener if desired. Cover with a lid and simmer gently on a low heat until the fruit becomes soft and the juice runs. Place the mixture in a food processor and liquidise or, alternatively, rub the fruit through a sieve using a wooden spoon.

Allow the purée to cool and place in a shallow container. Cover with cling film or foil and place in the freezer or the deep-freeze compartment of the refrigerator until the purée begins to set and crystallise. Remove the mixture from the freezer and stir it to form a soft crystallised consistency.

Whisk the 2 egg whites until they are stiff and

standing in peaks. Fold into the semi-frozen purée to give a marbled effect. Immediately return the mixture to the freezer and freeze until firm. Store in the freezer until required.

Remove from the freezer and place in the refrigerator 30 minutes before serving. Serve with fresh strawberries.

## Strawberry Wine Jelly

### SERVES 4

225g (8oz) fresh or frozen strawberries
2 tablespoons brandy
475ml (16fl oz) rosé wine
1 tablespoon powdered gelatine dissolved in 3 tablespoons hot water
2 tablespoons Canderel

*to decorate*
a few fresh strawberry leaves
4 whole strawberries

If using fresh strawberries, hull them first. Place the strawberries in a bowl and sprinkle on the brandy. Leave for 30 minutes, then pour the wine over and stir in the gelatine and Canderel.

Pour a little of the rosé wine and fruit into 4 serving glasses and leave to set in the refrigerator.

When set, add more of the wine and fruit and leave to set again. Continue to add the wine and fruit until it is all used up. This way, the fruit is suspended throughout the glass. Chill until set.

Decorate with strawberry leaves and strawberries.

## *Summer Delight*

SERVES 2

1 × 150g (5oz) fruit-flavoured diet yogurt
600ml (1 pint) jelly, made up with water
115g (4oz) low-fat cottage cheese
225g (8oz) fresh fruit of your choice
50g (2oz) Wall's 'Too Good To Be True' ice cream

Spoon alternate layers of yogurt, jelly, cottage cheese, fruit and ice cream into 2 large sundae glasses.

Garnish with some extra fruit and serve immediately.

## *Summer Pudding*

SERVES 6

Any selection of summer fruits can be used. Raspberries, redcurrants and blackcurrants are ideal, but take care not to use more than approximately 175g (6oz) of blackcurrants or their flavour will become too dominant. Blackberries, gooseberries, red cherries, red plums and strawberries can also be used. Stone cherries and plums and cut each plum half into 3–4 pieces. Cut large strawberries into quarters; leave the small ones whole.

Use day-old bread for this pudding. Cut it about as thick as you would for sandwiches. Baker's bread is better than sliced prepacked bread.

8–10 thin slices bread
675g (1½lb) soft fruit
115g (4oz) sugar

*to serve*
low-fat fromage frais

Cut the crusts from the bread and from one slice cut a circle about 25cm (1in) wider than the base of a 900ml (1½ pint) pudding basin. Reserve 1–2 slices to cover the top and cut the remainder of the bread into wedge shapes. Place the circle of bread in the base of the basin and arrange the wedge shapes around the side, making sure that they overlap in all places. If there should be a small gap anywhere, patch it on the inside with a small piece of bread. If you prefer, just line the inside of the basin with the slices of bread, rather than wedges. You will not waste any bread this way but it will look slightly less attractive.

Prepare the fruit as described and place the black-currants, redcurrants, blackberries, gooseberries, cherries and plums (according to the selection used) in a pan with the sugar and 150ml (¼ pint) water. Bring to the boil and simmer for 2–3 minutes. Add the raspberries and cook for a further minute. Add the strawberries, if used, and remove from the heat. It is not necessary to cook the fruit until it is soft, only until the sugar has dissolved and the juices are running from the fruit. With a slotted spoon, remove the fruit from the syrup and place in the prepared basin with sufficient syrup to moisten the bread. Reserve the remainder of the syrup. Place a piece of food wrap over the pudding and put a lightly weigh-ted saucer on top. Refrigerate overnight or for at least 6–8 hours.

Turn out the pudding carefully on to a serving dish. If any parts of the bread have not been saturated by the syrup, spoon a little of the reserved syrup over. Serve the rest separately, together with a bowl of low-fat fromage frais.

## Tiramisu

### SERVES 4 – 6

2 heaped teaspoons coffee granules or powder
2 teaspoons brandy
1 packet sponge fingers (approximately 12 fingers)
1 sachet Bird's Sugar-free Dream Topping
150ml (¼ pint) skimmed or semi-skimmed milk in addition to allowance
350g (12oz) low-fat fromage frais

*to serve*
powdered drinking chocolate

Mix the coffee with the brandy and make up to 150ml (¼ pint) with water.

Reserve half the sponge fingers and dip the remainder in the brandied coffee. Arrange the brandied fingers in the base of a serving dish to form a layer.

Make up the Dream Topping with the milk and mix in the fromage frais. Spoon half the mixture over the sponge fingers in the dish.

Dip the reserved sponge fingers in the remaining brandied coffee and place over the mixture in the dish.

Top with the remaining fromage frais mix. Sprinkle

with a little powdered drinking chocolate just before serving.

## Upside Down Fruit Meringue

### SERVES 2

1 × 60g (2¼oz) Marks and Spencer Low Fat Mousse
2 meringue nests
2 teaspoons cereal (e.g. muesli), crushed
1 peach or banana, sliced

Divide the mousse equally between the meringue nests and sprinkle each with 1 teaspoon of cereal. Decorate each with the sliced fruit.

## CAKES AND LOAVES

## Wholemeal Fruit Slice

### MAKES 16 × 1cm (½in) SLICES

1 teaspoon baking powder
115g (4oz) wholemeal flour
175g (6oz) mixed dried fruit or sultanas
75g (3oz) chopped dates
50g (2oz) bran
75g (3oz) chopped apricots
250ml (8fl oz) non-fat milk in addition to allowance

Preheat the oven to 160°C, 325°F or Gas mark 3.
 Combine all the ingredients in a bowl, then pour into a non-stick sponge roll tin. Press well down and bake in the oven for 35 minutes.

234

Allow to cool slightly and cut into slices while still warm.

## *Apricot Bread*

1 SERVING = 1cm (½in) SLICE

400g (14oz) plain flour
175g (6oz) sugar
½ teaspoon salt
1½ teaspoons baking powder
½ teaspoon bicarbonate of soda
75g (3oz) raisins or flaked almonds
175g (6oz) ready-to-eat or dried apricots, cut small and soaked in a little water
25g (1oz) butter
1 egg, beaten
grated rind and juice of 1 orange made up to 1 cup of liquid with more juice or Quosh

Preheat the oven to 180°C, 350°F or Gas mark 4.

Sift the flour, sugar, salt, baking powder and bicarbonate of soda into a large bowl. Add the raisins or almonds and apricots and mix well.

Melt the butter. Make a well in the centre of the mixture. Add the butter, egg, grated rind and juice and stir into the mixture.

Place in a 900g (2lb) loaf tin and bake in the oven for 50–60 minutes.

Remove from the oven and leave to cool. When cool, place in an airtight container and keep for 24 hours before using.

# Bran Loaf

1 SERVING = 1cm ($\frac{1}{2}$in) SLICE

1 cup branflakes or All-Bran
1 cup sultanas
1 cup skimmed or semi-skimmed milk in addition to
allowance
$\frac{1}{2}$ cup brown sugar
pinch of mixed spice (optional)
1 cup wholemeal self-raising flour

Place all the ingredients except the flour in a bowl and leave for 1 hour.

Preheat the oven to 160°C, 325°F or Gas mark 3.

Add the flour and stir well. Place in a greased and base-lined 450g (1lb) loaf tin and bake in the oven for 1 hour 10 minutes.

Remove from the oven and turn out on to a wire rack to cool.

# *Carrot Cake*

## MAKES 10 SLICES

275g (10oz) soft light brown sugar
1 large can prunes, stoned and puréed
grated rind of 1 orange
4 eggs
400g (14oz) self-raising flour
2 teaspoons baking powder
1 teaspoon bicarbonate of soda
1 teaspoon ground ginger
1 teaspoon mixed spice
1 teaspoon ground nutmeg
450g (1lb) carrots, peeled and finely grated
175g (6oz) sultanas

Preheat the oven to 180°C, 350°F or Gas mark 4. Lightly grease and line a 25cm (10in) round cake tin.

In a large bowl, cream together the sugar, puréed prunes and orange rind until light and fluffy. Gradually beat in the eggs.

Fold in the flour and the remaining dry ingredients, a little at a time.

Finally, fold in the grated carrots and sultanas. If the mixture seems a little too stiff, slacken it with a drop of milk.

Transfer into the prepared tin and bake in the oven for 1–1¼ hours. Leave to cool in the tin.

# Carrot and Ginger Cake

### MAKES 8-10 1cm (½in) SLICES

225g (8oz) self-raising flour
175g (6oz) dark brown soft sugar
2 teaspoons ground ginger
2 large carrots, grated
1 egg, beaten
250ml (8fl oz) skimmed or semi-skimmed milk

Preheat the oven to 180°C, 350°F or Gas mark 4. Line a 450g (1lb) tin with greaseproof paper or use a non-stick tin.

Mix the flour, sugar and ground ginger in a bowl. Add the grated carrots and stir well. Add the beaten egg to the milk. Stir into the mixture and mix well.

Pour the mixture into the prepared tin and bake in the oven for 50–55 minutes, until a skewer inserted into the cake comes out clean.

Leave to cool. When the cake is quite cool, remove the paper and place in an airtight tin to store.

# Malt Loaf

### 1 SERVING = 1cm (½in) SLICE

1 cup bran
1 cup mixed dried fruit or sultanas
1 cup muscovado sugar
1 cup skimmed or semi-skimmed milk
1 cup self-raising flour

Line a 450g (1lb) loaf tin with greaseproof paper.

Mix together the bran, mixed fruit or sultanas, sugar and milk and leave to stand for 1 hour.

Preheat the oven to 160°C, 320°F or Gas mark 3.

Sieve the flour, then mix into the other ingredients. Pour into the loaf tin and bake in the oven for about 1 hour.

Remove from the oven and allow to cool.

## *Marmalade Cake*

1 SERVING = 1 cm ($\frac{1}{2}$in) SLICE

225g (8oz) mixed dried fruit
1 mug cold tea
225g (8oz) self-raising flour
115g (4oz) caster sugar
1 egg, beaten
2 tablespoons marmalade

Soak the mixed fruit in the tea overnight until the fruit swells.

Preheat the oven to 180°C, 350°F or Gas mark 4.

In a bowl combine the flour, sugar, egg and marmalade, then add the fruit mix. Mix well and place in a lined or non-stick 675g (1½lb) loaf tin and bake in oven for 1 hour.

Leave to cool before slicing.

## Moist Fruit Cake

### MAKES 18 SERVINGS

250ml (8fl oz) non-fat milk
50g (2oz) brown sugar
1 tablespoon Golden Syrup
1 banana, mashed
450g (1lb) fruit mix
1 teaspoon vanilla
175g (6oz) plain flour
1 teaspoon baking powder
1 teaspoon cinnamon
1 teaspoon ginger

*for the icing*
lemon essence
vanilla essence
almond essence

Mix together the milk, sugar, Golden Syrup, banana, fruit mix and vanilla and leave to soak for 1 hour.

Preheat the oven to 160°C, 325°F or Gas mark 3. Line a Swiss roll or cake tin with greaseproof paper.

Sieve the flour, baking powder, cinnamon and ginger into a bowl then stir it into the wet mixture.

Transfer the mixture into the Swiss roll or cake tin and bake in the oven for 45–60 minutes. To test whether the cake is cooked, insert a skewer in the centre of the cake. The skewer should come out dry.

Leave to cool. When cold, mix together the icing

ingredients with a little water and smooth evenly on top of the cake.

## *Sultana Loaf*

1 SERVING = 1cm (¹/₂in) SLICE

225g (8oz) self-raising flour
1¹/₂ teaspoons mixed spice
1¹/₂ teaspoons cinnamon
75g (3oz) brown sugar
350g (12oz) sultanas
300ml (¹/₂ pint) non-fat milk or soya milk

Preheat the oven to 160°C, 325°F or Gas mark 3.

Mix together the flour, mixed spice and cinnamon and add the sugar and sultanas. Add the milk and mix to make a soft dough.

Pour the mixture into a loaf tin lined with grease-proof paper, and bake in the oven for approximately 1 hour.

## *Weetabix Cake*

1 SERVING = 0.5cm (¹/₄in) SLICE

2 Weetabix
300ml (¹/₂ pint) skimmed or semi-skimmed milk
225g (8oz) soft brown sugar
225g (8oz) mixed dried fruit
1 egg, beaten
225g (8oz) self-raising flour

Place the Weetabix, milk, brown sugar and dried fruit into a mixing bowl and leave to soak in the fridge overnight.

Preheat the oven to 180°C, 350°F or Gas Mark 4.

Add the beaten egg and flour to the mixture and mix thoroughly. Transfer to a lined 900g (2lb) loaf tin. Bake in the oven for 1¼ hours until well risen and golden brown. To test whether the cake is cooked, insert a skewer into the centre of the cake. The skewer should come out clean.

# Sauces and Dressings

## Citrus Dressing

120ml (4fl oz) fresh orange juice
50ml (2fl oz) lemon juice
50ml (2fl oz) wine vinegar
1 teaspoon Dijon mustard
salt and pepper

Place all the ingredients in a clean screw-top jar and shake well. Keep in the refrigerator and use within 3 days.

# Oil-free Vinaigrette Dressing

3 tablespoons white wine vinegar or cider vinegar
1 tablespoon lemon juice
1½ teaspoon black pepper
½ teaspoon salt
1 teaspoon sugar
½ teaspoon French mustard
chopped herbs (thyme, marjoram, basil or parsley)

Mix all the ingredients together. Place in a container, seal and shake well. Taste and add more salt or sugar as desired. Keep in the refrigerator and use within 3 days.

# Reduced-Oil Dressing

3 tablespoons reduced-oil, low-calorie salad dressing (any brand)
1 × 150g (5oz) carton diet yogurt
salt and pepper to taste

Mix all the ingredients in a container. Keep in the refrigerator and use within 2 days.

# Seafood Dressing

### MAKES 2 SERVINGS

1 tablespoon tomato ketchup
1 tablespoon reduced-oil salad dressing (e.g. Waistline)
4 tablespoons low-fat natural yogurt
a dash of Tabasco sauce
salt and pepper to taste

Mix all the ingredients together in a container and store in the refrigerator. Use within 2 days.

# Yogurt Dressing

150g (5oz) low-fat natural yogurt
a good squeeze of lemon juice
salt and freshly ground black pepper to taste

Mix all the ingredients together in a container and store in the refrigerator for up to 2 days. As a variation, add $\frac{1}{2}$ teaspoon prepared mint sauce.

# Yogurt and Mint Dressing

150g (5oz) low-fat natural yogurt
1 teaspoon mint sauce
salt and freshly ground black pepper to taste

Mix all the ingredients together in a container. Store in the refrigerator and use within 2 days.

# Garlic and Mint Yogurt Dip

### SERVES 4

150g (5oz) low-fat natural yogurt
1 clove garlic, peeled and finely chopped
2 sprigs fresh mint, chopped
115g (4oz) low-fat cottage cheese

Mix all the ingredients together. Serve in a small dish and use as a dip for crudités.

# *Barbecue Sauce*

## MAKES 2 SERVINGS

3 tablespoons tomato ketchup
3 tablespoons brown sauce
1 teaspoon mustard
2 tablespoons garlic and chilli sauce
6 tablespoons tomato juice
1 clove garlic, peeled and crushed (optional)
freshly ground black pepper

Mix all the ingredients together and brush on to meat, chicken or fish kebabs, preferably an hour or two before cooking. Heat any remaining sauce and serve separately.

# *Cocktail Sauce*

*allow the following amounts per person*
1 tablespoon tomato ketchup
$\frac{1}{2}$ teaspoon reduced-oil, low-calorie salad dressing (any brand)
freshly ground black pepper to taste
a dash of Tabasco sauce
1 tablespoon low-fat natural yogurt

Mix all the ingredients together in a container and store in a refrigerator until needed. Use within 2 days.

# *Parsley Sauce*

## SERVES 4

300ml (½ pint) skimmed or semi-skimmed milk
1 onion, peeled and sliced
6 peppercorns
1 bay leaf
salt and black pepper
2 teaspoons cornflour
chopped fresh parsley

Gently heat all but 50ml (2fl oz) of the milk in a non-stick saucepan. Add the onion, peppercorns, bay leaf, salt and pepper. Cover the pan and simmer for 5 minutes. Turn off the heat and leave the milk to stand with the lid on for a further 30 minutes or until it is time to thicken and serve the sauce.

Mix the remaining milk with the cornflour, and when almost time to serve, strain the infused milk, add the cornflour mixture and reheat slowly, stirring continuously, until the mixture comes to the boil. Add the chopped parsley. If the sauce begins to thicken too quickly, remove from the heat and stir very fast to mix well. Cook for 3–4 minutes and serve immediately.

# 8

---

# Exercise Your Way to a Flatter Stomach

Nature has given us the most magnificent, built-in, natural girdle in the form of our abdominal and back muscles, which work in conjunction with each other to help maintain a good posture. There are four major muscle groups in the abdomen. We have a band of horizontal muscle (the transversus muscle) across our abdominal area, and we use this muscle each time we hold our tummy in. On top of this band are a pair of diagonal strips of muscle (the internal and external obliques) which define the waistline. And reaching from the lower part of the ribcage down to the pubic bone is a strip of muscle (the rectus abdominus) just waiting to show off a lovely flat tum.

As we gain weight, these muscles become disguised under the flab and their ability to display a good body shape is lost. Once we gain a lot of fat around our abdominal area, no amount of holding our tummy in is going to make that fat disappear. Eventually, we simply give up trying to hold ourselves well and just let it all hang out! The result is that the muscles weaken through lack of use. But just because your muscles are underused now does not mean they have to stay that way, just as the fat sitting on your stomach doesn't have to stay there for ever either. In this chapter I will show you how you can burn the fat, find your muscles again and have a stomach that you can be proud of.

## Getting rid of the fat

We know that any excess food in our diet is stored on the body as fat. It's as if the fat we eat has a direct motorway link to our fat deposit boxes (fat cells) on the abdomen, hips and thighs. It is easy to understand therefore that if we use up some of those stores of fat by increasing our energy output through exercise and at the same time do not replace those fat stores by consuming vast quantities of fat, the amount of fat on the body will dramatically reduce. This fact has been proved beyond doubt by the evidence of my trial team and the hundreds of thousands of people who have successfully slimmed on my diets.

There are two main types of exercise that will help us in our flat stomach campaign. Both are immensely valuable in our war against fat but they serve quite different purposes. The first is aerobic exercise, which burns fat, and the second is commonly called toning or strengthening exercise, which works specific muscle groups. The second type of exercise helps to build muscle which, in turn, increases the metabolic rate – the rate at which we burn calories – since muscle requires energy to sustain it. If you want to enjoy the benefits of having a flatter stomach, you need to undertake both types of exercise.

## Aerobic exercise

The word 'aerobic' literally means 'with oxygen' and is used to describe any exercise which causes the heart and lungs to work harder as the body demands a greater intake of oxygen to supply the energy to sustain the activity. Aerobic exercise, therefore, is any activity that makes you puff a bit. Once the body has warmed up, its capacity to continue with aerobic exercise is remarkable. For instance, you could go for a moderately brisk walk and walk several miles without becoming too exhausted because you would be breathing in oxygen which would be supplying you with enough fuel to keep you going. Providing you had sufficient oxygen circulating in your bloodstream, then you could keep going almost indefinitely. The only reason you would want to stop is because your feet were sore, not because your heart and lungs couldn't take it. But you don't have to go on a ten-mile hike to enjoy the benefits of aerobic exercise.

All exercise causes us to use extra calories, and that's good news for anyone trying to lose weight. The more active you are, the more weight you will lose. If you do aerobic exercise, then you will actually be burning fat calories. Cycling (indoors or outdoors), brisk walking, jogging, swimming or exercising on a rowing machine are all aerobic activities and will burn fat off your body. The ideal is to do 10–15 minutes of aerobic exercise five days a week. Just as a car burns petrol, so your body will call upon its stores of fat as an energy source. If you don't believe me, just look at any long-distance runner and see how lean they are.

If you're thinking that you haven't got time to exercise five times a week, then ask yourself how badly you want to be slim. One of the trial dieters commented: 'Before I started this diet I couldn't find time to exercise, but now I *make* time. It is so worthwhile and has made all the difference to my body shape.' Some people prefer to exercise first thing in the morning and get up early in order to do so – I certainly prefer to exercise at this time of day – while others find it more convenient in the evening. It doesn't matter *when* you exercise, as long as you do it. If you can exercise with others, then so much the better, because you will encourage each other and are more likely to keep it up. Keep a record of your activity (see page 335).

## Toning or strengthening exercise

Toning exercise will help build and strengthen our muscles to give us a better body shape. Muscle is an active tissue which requires fuel (calories) to sustain it, therefore the more muscle you have, the more calories you will burn and the higher your metabolic rate will be. On a low-fat, calorie-controlled diet of around 1,400 calories a day, as this diet is, you will lose mostly fat from your body, but inevitably you will also lose a tiny amount of muscle tissue. This is why crash diets are so unhealthy. Very low calorie diets make the body believe it is starving. To prevent starvation, therefore, the body stores the food that you do eat as fat and uses lean muscle tissue as an energy source. This causes the metabolic rate to fall so that once you return to 'normal' eating, you inevitably gain weight. It is essential, therefore, that anyone who goes on a weight-loss diet eats sufficient calories to prevent a dramatic reduction in muscle tissue and also takes regular exercise to maintain their muscle mass.

In this programme we will be focusing on the abdominal and back muscles, which work together to give us a better posture and muscle balance. When we work a muscle, it becomes stronger and tighter. Therefore, if we were to work only the abdominal muscles, over a period of time, our posture might suffer and we could begin to slump forwards. That's why it is equally important to work the muscles in the back to provide a counter-balance and enable us to remain upright in a good posture.

Furthermore, if we are to increase our muscle mass, we need to challenge the muscle to work a little harder than it is currently used to working. You should aim to perform sufficient repetitions to enable the muscle to become mildly fatigued and then do two more repetitions to challenge it further – but not strain it. Challenging the muscle in this way will enable it to increase in strength and size.

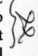

However, the exercise programme in this book is

not designed to give you muscles like Arnold Schwarzenegger. To achieve such massive muscles you would need to work with increasingly heavy weights to encourage a very concentrated development of the muscles. This is why weight-lifters who want to dramatically increase their muscle bulk work to a maximum level of weight resistance with a low number of repetitions. Their energy is concentrated in short, sharp bursts, and therefore they don't require the same level of stamina that is required for aerobic exercise. With the programme in this book we work with light to moderate weight which means you can achieve excellent toning of the muscle without adding bulk.

## Exercise for health

Exercise, combined with diet, will help us to achieve the optimum progress in our weight-loss campaign, but there are many additional benefits to be gained from exercise. Studies have shown that people who combine diet and exercise are likely to be much more successful in keeping the weight off in the long term.

Most people are aware that the heart and lungs benefit from aerobic exercise. We can more than halve our risk of heart disease if we exercise regularly. There are many other advantages to health, some of which are particularly important for women. Osteoporosis, otherwise known as brittle bone disease, affects one in three older women, and regular exercise can be of enormous help in preventing this condition. All the exercises described in this book will help achieve this aim. The ideal way is to combine aerobic exercise, such as brisk walking, with some toning or strength work for the muscles in order to encourage the maintenance of bone density.

Exercise can also help reduce stress and anxiety as well as increase our energy levels and enable us to enjoy life to the full. The benefits are to all people of all ages, and it's never too late to start. Recent trials have shown that even those people who are well advanced in years can achieve a marked improvement in the quality of life by becoming more active.

It is important to realise that exercise can mean any form of physical activity. You don't have to go to a formal exercise class or spend half an hour on a rowing machine to feel that you have worked out. The key is to increase the amount of activity in your daily life. You can choose to do this in one long session each day or incorporate it into lots of little sessions. So, for instance, you could go and play football with the children for half an hour, or you could fit in little snippets of activity around your everyday tasks. Park your car at the furthest spot, not the nearest, when you go to the supermarket; take the stairs, not the lift; mow the lawn or dig the garden when you come home from work; walk or cycle to work instead of taking the car, bus or train. A policeman I met recently told me that he had lost half a stone simply because he had stopped accepting a lift to work and instead did the 15-minute walk from his house to the station. This small lifestyle change had made a real difference to his weight.

Exercise should therefore become a habit and form

part of our everyday lifestyle. Once we make the effort, it becomes a way of life, and that is the best insurance policy we can give ourselves.

# The complete flat stomach plan workout

The exercise plan that follows is designed to offer a comprehensive programme that suits all levels of ability and specifically targets the abdominal area. The routines are arranged in three different levels: Elementary, Intermediate and Advanced.

It is a good idea to start with the Elementary routine as this teaches you the basics of correct abdominal technique with the Pelvic Tilt.

You will find that each routine also includes some work for the spine and the postural muscles at the back of the shoulders. This ensures a balanced programme that will develop and tone all the muscles in the trunk to make a real difference in the way you look and hold yourself.

Each time you work out, always start by loosening up with the recommended warm-up exercises on pages 256–262. These will raise the body temperature and prepare your muscles and joints for the work they are about to undertake, thereby increasing the effectiveness of the exercises that follow. If you omit the warm-up exercises, then you run a risk of injury and the exercises will not be as beneficial. Raising the body temperature even slightly goes a long way to improving performance.

Always finish your workout with the cool-down stretches on pages 276–279 to enable your muscles to return to normal and prevent any aches or pains later.

Once you feel ready to move on to the next level, always begin with just a few repetitions of each new toning exercise and gradually increase the number until you can comfortably cope. Working a muscle too hard too soon runs the risk of damaging the muscle and makes the experience of exercise painful. This alone can deter you from practising regularly. Although each exercise should cause some discomfort in order to provide sufficient challenge, you should not feel any pain.

Practise these exercises as often as you can, every day if possible, since consistency is important if you are to see genuine results. Lack of time is a common excuse for not being consistent with an exercise programme, but each of these routines takes only ten minutes. So, you could set your alarm clock ten minutes earlier and do your workout as soon as you get out of bed in the morning so that it becomes a habit. Any time of day is acceptable, but if you set aside the same period of time each day, then you are far more likely to stick with it.

## The Warm-up

Just as we would warm up our Plasticene or Play-doh before we used it, we need to warm up by mobilising the joints then warming and stretching the muscles before exercise. Neglecting to do so could cause serious damage which could take weeks to repair. Also, by warming up thoroughly we increase the heart rate and flow of blood around the body. As a result, the muscles work harder and therefore derive more benefit from the workout. It only takes a few minutes to warm up and it is a great investment towards a fitter body. Do this short section before each workout.

### Posture check

First check your posture. Good posture is essential if you are to achieve a flat stomach, and it will also improve your overall health and wellbeing. So get into good posture habits.

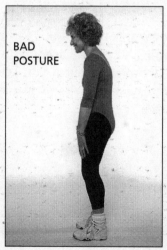

BAD POSTURE

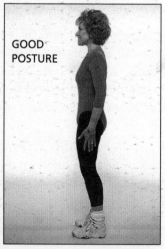

GOOD POSTURE

Stand as tall as you can, pulling your tummy in and taking your shoulders back and down. Your shoulders should be in line with your ankles. Try to adopt this posture at all times. It's one of the best things you can do for your figure. Look in the mirror and see what a difference it makes.

Now let's move on to the warm-up exercises.

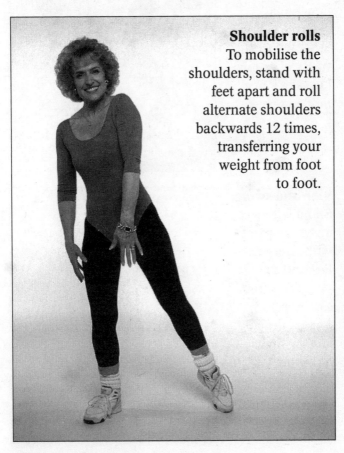

**Shoulder rolls**
To mobilise the shoulders, stand with feet apart and roll alternate shoulders backwards 12 times, transferring your weight from foot to foot.

### Ski down

Maintaining a good posture with tummy pulled in tightly, swing both arms up and down, bending your knees as you lower the arms. Do 16 swings up and down in a smooth, skiing motion. Do not rush the action but take it at a moderate pace.

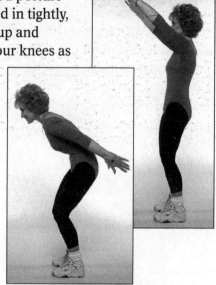

### Step and swing

Stand with feet apart. Step out with alternate feet and swing your arms from side to side. Repeat the step and swinging movement 20 times (10 each side).

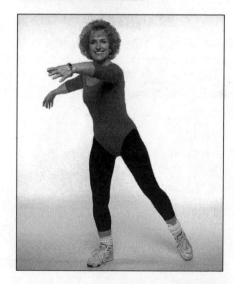

## Side bends

Stand with feet hip-width apart, knees slightly bent and hands on hips. Keep your hips facing forwards and slowly lean to the side, reaching out with your arm. Straighten up and repeat to the other side. Repeat 8 times to alternate sides (4 each side).

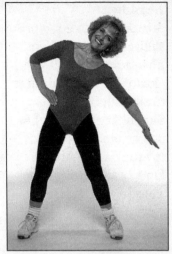

## Opposite hand to knee

Maintaining a good posture with your back straight, raise alternate knees across the body and swing and touch with alternate hands. Do 24 (12 each knee). Try not to bend forwards as you raise the knee.

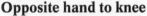

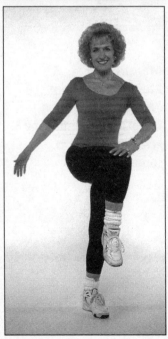

**Waist twist**
Stand with knees
slightly apart and bent,
hips facing straight
ahead and arms raised
to shoulder level.
Slowly twist your upper
body from side to side
to mobilise the spine.
Do 8 twists to alternate
sides (4 each side).

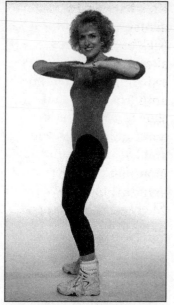

**Marching**
March on the spot,
swinging your arms
freely and maintaining a
good posture. Do 32
steps.

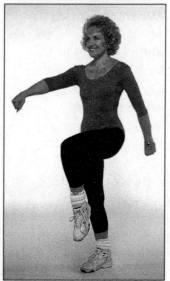

## Kick back, swing across

Kick back with alternate feet, swinging your arms from side to side. Work up a good momentum and keep the movement smooth and rhythmic. Do 24 steps (12 each side).

Now do your stretches.

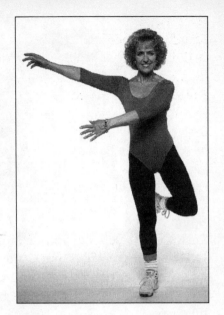

## Warm-up Stretches

### Waist stretch

Sit on the floor with legs crossed and place one hand on the floor for support. Reach over to the side with the other arm, palm facing upwards, and hold for 10 seconds. Repeat to the other side.

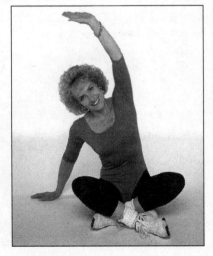

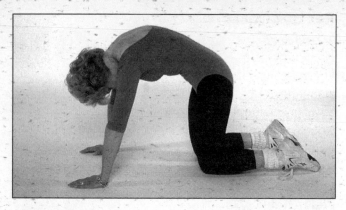

**Spine stretch**

Position yourself on your hands and knees, with knees under your hips and hands under your shoulders. Pull your tummy right into your spine and arch your back as much as possible. Hold for 6 seconds, then relax.

If you find kneeling uncomfortable, practise the spine stretch from the cool-down (see page 277).

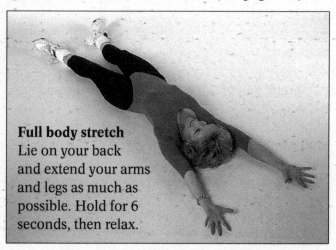

**Full body stretch**
Lie on your back and extend your arms and legs as much as possible. Hold for 6 seconds, then relax.

## Routine One: Elementary

Remember always to do the warm-up sequence on pages 256–62 before you start the following exercises.

### Pelvic tilt

Learning to tilt your pelvis correctly is important if you are to perform the abdominal exercises properly and effectively. So make sure you have mastered this tilt before you move on to the following exercises.

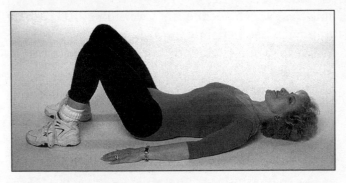

Lie on your back, bend your knees and rest your hands on the floor by your sides.

Press your lower spine into the floor and gently tilt your pelvis, easing your hips slightly towards your ribcage. Release. The movement is slight and your spine should always remain on the floor.

Do 12 pelvic tilts to practise, and remember to incorporate this movement in every abdominal exercise.

### Waist tightener

This elementary exercise is easy to do and is a good way to start toning and strengthening the oblique

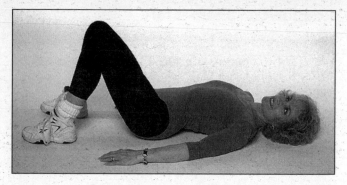

muscles which define the waistline. Keep your tummy pulled in tightly throughout.

Lie on your back with knees bent and arms by your sides.

Slowly curve your left hip towards your left shoulder, then return to the central position. Now, curve your right hip towards your right shoulder then straighten again. Perform this slowly and rhythmically.

Do 16 hip shifts to alternate sides (8 each side).

## Abdominal curl

Lie on your back with knees bent. Place one hand behind your head to support it and place the other

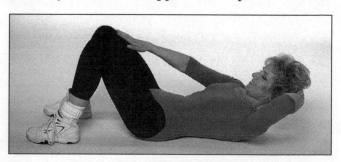

arm on your thigh. Pull your tummy in tightly and feel your spine in contact with the floor.

Slowly raise your head and shoulders a few inches off the floor, keeping your chin away from your chest and allowing your outstretched hand to move up your thigh towards your knee. Slowly lower your head and shoulders back to the floor. Move slowly and rhythmically, breathing out as you come up and breathing in as you lower.

Repeat 8 times, then rest and repeat if possible.

## Back strengthener

Lie face down, bend your elbows and position them close by your sides with your palms down.

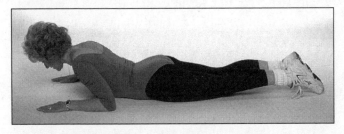

Using the strength in your back, slowly raise your head and shoulders, then lower them again. Always look towards the floor.

Repeat 6 times if possible. Build up the number of repetitions as your back becomes stronger, but do not strain.

## Waist trimmer

Lie on your back with knees bent. Place your right hand behind your head for support and the other arm by your side.

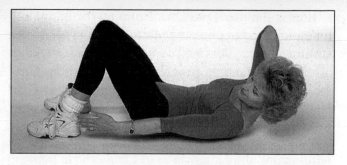

Slowly curve your body to the left and reach your left hand towards your left foot to work the waist muscles on your left side. Slowly return to the central position, switch the position of your hands and repeat to the other side.

Do 16 curves to alternate sides (8 each side), keeping your tummy pulled in tight throughout. Rest and repeat if possible.

## Back strengthener

Lie face down, bend your elbows and position them close to your sides, this time with palms up.

Using the strength of your back, not your arms, slowly raise your head and shoulders, then lower them again.

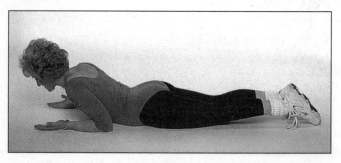

Repeat 8 times if possible. Build up the number of repetitions as your back becomes stronger but do not strain.

To prevent muscle soreness and return your body to its natural state do the cool-down stretches on pages 276–78.

When you feel confident that Routine One is well within your ability, move on to the more challenging Intermediate workout that follows.

## Routine Two: Intermediate

For maximum benefit, don't attempt this routine until you can complete Routine One comfortably.

Remember always to do the warm-up routine on pages 256–62 before you commence this workout.

### Abdominal curl

Lie on your back with knees bent and legs resting on a chair. Place your arms across your chest.

Pulling your tummy in tightly, slowly raise your head and shoulders off the floor. Make sure you keep

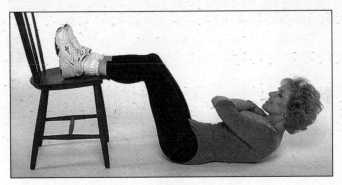

your chin away from your chest. Breathe out as you raise and breathe in as you lower.

Repeat 8 times, rest and repeat. If your neck begins to ache, place one hand behind your head for support.

## Posture improver
Our lifestyles encourage us to slump forwards, leaving us with round shoulders. This exercise, if practised regularly, will help counteract this problem.

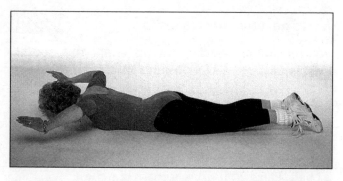

Lie face down, bend your arms and position your elbows at shoulder level. Slowly raise your bent arms as if trying to bring your shoulder blades together, then lower them again.

Repeat 8 times or to the point of mild discomfort.

## Waist toner
Lie on your back with knees bent and your legs resting on a chair. Place one hand behind your head and rest your elbow on the floor for support.

Pull your tummy in tightly, then slowly raise and twist your upper body and reach your arm across

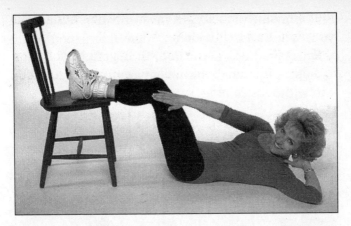

towards the opposite knee. Slowly lower your body
to the floor. Breath out as you lift and in as you lower.

Repeat 8 times, then switch arms and repeat to the
other side. Rest and repeat if possible.

**Back strengthener**

If you have practised the back strengthening exercises in Routine One, you may be able to progress to
this more advanced version. If you find it too challenging, go back to one of the easier versions in Routine One.

Lie face down with your hands by your sides,
palms up.

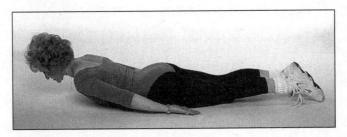

Using only the strength in your back, slowly raise your head and shoulders off the floor, then lower them again. Look at the floor throughout.

Repeat this small movement as many times as you can without straining.

### Reverse curl

Lie on your back with knees bent and arms out at your sides. Raise your legs so that your feet are above your hips, and cross your ankles.

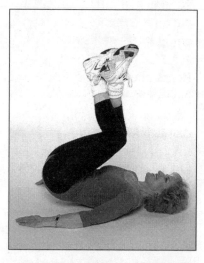

Pull your tummy in tightly and press your spine into the floor. Using your abdominal muscles, try to lift your hips towards the ceiling, then lower them again. Keep the movement smooth and try not to rock your body. Make sure you use only the strength in your abdomen – even the smallest of movements is valuable.

Repeat 8 times if possible. Rest and repeat.

Repeat Routine Two once more, then move on to the cool-down stretches on pages 276–78.

When you can perform this Intermediate workout with ease, move on to the Advanced workout in Routine Three.

## Routine Three: Advanced

This is an advanced workout and should only be attempted when you find the Intermediate workout insufficiently challenging. Remember, you only need to feel mild discomfort for an exercise to be effective. To reach a point of pain would be a signal that damage is being done. So listen to your body and enjoy the benefits of this advanced workout.

Remember always to do the warm-up routine on pages 256–62 before you start.

### Abdominal curl
Lie on your back with knees bent, tummy pulled in tightly and spine in contact with the floor. Place your hands to either side of your head.

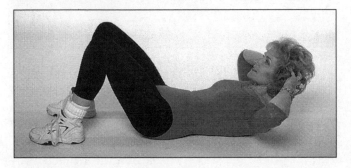

Slowly raise your head and shoulders off the floor, keeping your chin away from your chest, then lower your head and shoulders to the floor again. Breathe out as you raise and breathe in as you lower.

Repeat as many times as you can until you feel some mild discomfort. Rest and repeat.

## Opposite arm and leg lift

Lie face down on the floor with arms and legs extended.

Raise your left arm and right leg simultaneously, keeping them straight, then lower them again. Repeat with the right arm and left leg. Keep the lifting movement smooth and controlled.

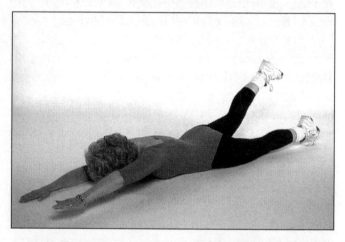

Only do as many repetitions as you comfortably can. Try 3 repetitions on each side at first and gradually increase the number as you become stronger.

## Waist twister

Lie on your back with knees bent and place your hands to either side of your head. Raise your left leg and rest it across the front of the right leg.

Slowly raise your head and shoulders and twist your upper body, lifting your right shoulder towards your left knee, resting your left elbow on the floor for support. Slowly lower your upper body to the floor.

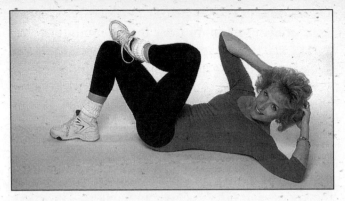

Breathe out as you raise and breathe in as you lower and keep your tummy pulled in throughout.

Repeat 8 times, then switch the position of the arms and legs and repeat to the other side. Rest, then do 8 more repetitions to each side.

**Back and shoulder strengthener**
Only attempt this exercise if you feel completely comfortable with the back strengthening exercises in Routines One and Two. Once you have reached this level of strength, practise your back exercises regularly to maintain your muscle strength, as this will stand you in good stead for years.

Lie face down on the floor and place your hands on your seat.

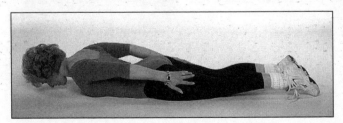

Pull your shoulder blades together, then slowly raise your upper body from the floor, and lower it again. Make sure you maintain good control, and keep looking at the floor throughout.

Repeat as many times as possible until you feel some mild discomfort.

## Waist shrinker

Lie on your back with knees bent. Slowly raise your knees and extend your legs above your hips, keeping the knees slightly bent. Cross your ankles. Place your left hand behind your head for support.

Pull your tummy in tightly, then lift your head and shoulders and aim to reach the right hand up and across your body towards the left foot, resting your left elbow on the floor for support. Slowly lower your head and shoulders to the floor.

Repeat, this time aiming your left hand towards your right foot. Keep alternating sides for a total count of 8. Rest and repeat.

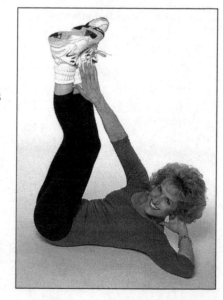

**Posture Improver**

Lie face down, bend your arms and position your elbows at shoulder level. Slowly raise your bent arms as if trying to bring your shoulder blades together, then lower them again.

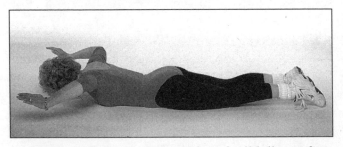

Repeat 10 times or to the point of mild discomfort.

**Crunch**

Lie on your back with knees bent and place your hands to either side of your head. Slowly raise your bent legs and cross them at the ankles.

Press your abdomen into your spine and slowly raise your head and shoulders, keeping the chin

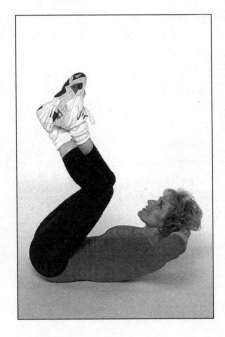

275

away from the chest. At the same time lift your legs towards the ceiling to slightly raise your hips off the floor. Breathe out as you raise and breathe in as you lower.

Repeat as many times as is comfortable, without straining. Rest and repeat.

Now do your cool-down stretches.

## Cool-Down Stretches

Each time you work your muscles quite hard it is important to stretch them out again afterwards to prevent soreness and bring them back to their natural state. So always finish your toning workout with these stretches. They should be performed slowly and held quite still in the extreme position. Perform them once only.

**Waist stretch**
Sit on the floor with your legs crossed and your torso upright. Place one hand on the floor for support and reach the other arm up and over your head. Hold for 10 seconds, then relax and repeat on the other side.

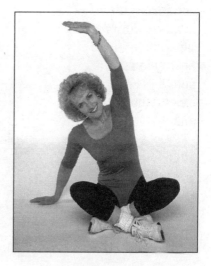

**Spine stretch**
Sitting cross-legged with tummy pulled in, curl the spine and extend your arms out on the floor in front. Hold for 10 seconds, then relax.

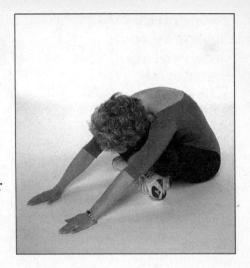

**Shoulder stretch**
Still sitting with legs crossed and tummy pulled in tightly, extend your arms forwards to stretch the shoulder area. Allow your head to drop forwards slightly. Hold for 10 seconds, then relax.

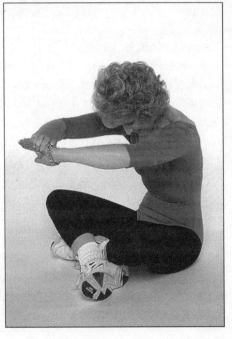

**Posture stretch**
Sitting in a good posture with legs crossed or in a relaxed position in front, extend both arms behind you. Hold this extended position for 10 seconds and feel the stretch in your chest area. Relax.

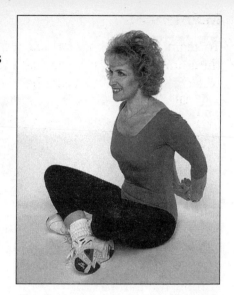

**Tummy stretch**
Lie face down on the floor. Bend your arms and position them so that the elbows are beneath the shoulders. Keeping your forearms and elbows on the floor, gently raise your head and shoulders and feel the stretch down the front of your abdominal area. Hold for 6 seconds, then relax.

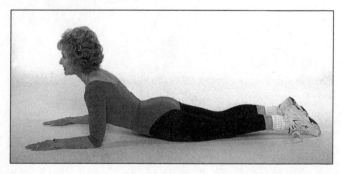

## Maintenance

To maintain the progress you
these toning exercises, practise
week. Feel free to alternate betwe
and Three in order to vary your w
easier to keep the muscle tone you h
to achieve in the first place, so make
on to it now!

I fully understand that it's not always easy to follow an exercise routine from a book. With this in mind, I have devised a Complete Flat Stomach Plan workout video to accompany this book. The video offers a wider selection of exercises to offer you greater variety and also includes a fun, fat-burning aerobic routine.

# 9

# Enjoy a Flat Stomach for Life

If you have followed this diet strictly and undertaken the exercises as recommended your stomach should now be significantly flatter. The challenge now is to maintain that progress and keep your stomach flat for good.

Now that you have successfully completed this Complete Flat Stomach Plan, your body will be familiar with the quantities of food that you have been feeding it. Over a period of time, your body will acclimatise to this level of intake and your rate of weight loss will inevitably slow down. Also, your body will not require as much energy to go about its everyday tasks since it now has less weight to carry around than before. When you reach your target weight, therefore, it is important that you increase your daily intake of food by a few hundred calories so that your body returns to 'normal' operation, doesn't feel it is dieting and maintains a healthy equilibrium between energy input and output.

All you need to do is to slightly increase the amount of food so that you are eating an extra 150 calories or so per day for the first week. This can be achieved by having an extra ounce of cereal or slice of toast for breakfast and an extra piece of fruit for lunch. The following week, increase your food intake by a further 100 calories or so by adding another piece of fruit for lunch and having an extra ounce of pasta or rice or an extra potato with your evening meal. Once you become confident that you can eat these additional amounts and not gain weight, you can then relax and not worry too much about quantities.

One word of warning, though. While you don't have to be quite so strict about your food intake, please do not return to your old, high-fat eating habits. If you start including vast quantities of oil, butter, cream and fat into your diet again you will be astonished at how quickly you will gain weight.

I learned this the hard way a couple of years ago when I was in Los Angeles filming a TV series. The salads in America are quite exceptional and I decided to enjoy the wonderful Caesar salad that the chef at the hotel prepared. I left the croûtons but, while I realised that the dressing would contain oil, I thought the amount would be insignificant. After all, I wasn't trying to lose weight, I was just trying to stay at my existing weight. How wrong I was. I was away for only seven days, but during that time I gained four pounds and it was definitely the oil that did it.

You can see how easy it is to convince ourselves that something is harmless because it looks innocuous. Oil and fat don't look much and you don't actually chew them, so you hardly notice they are there. Yet, they are singularly the most damaging foods as far as your figure is concerned. Avoid them whenever you can, and certainly don't start acquiring a taste for them again. You have broken your old, high-fat eating habits, so please keep it that way.

Keep up your new level of activity and enjoy the fact that you are so much slimmer and fitter now. Remember that every bit of activity you do is helping to keep you young and in shape. It's the most positive investment you can make.

## Ten Tips to Help You Maintain Your New Figure

1 Continue to eat three meals a day and don't skip breakfast. Try not to eat between meals, although you can now have the occasional piece of fruit between meals. If you find your weight creeping back up though, you will need to stop this habit.

2 Eat low-fat foods and observe the four per cent fat ruling on all foods you buy. If occasionally you fancy something with a higher fat content, by all means have it and enjoy it, but don't get into the habit of having butter on your bread or cream with your dessert. You have now re-educated your taste buds, but it wouldn't take too much to slip back into your old habits, and that's the last thing you want to do. Remember, the fat you eat is stored as fat on your body. Eat lean and you'll stay lean.

3 Always cook low fat, even when cooking for

others. Never return to the habit of cooking with oil or adding cream or butter to your dishes. You have broken these habits, please don't let them return.

4 Allow yourself the occasional treat. Don't get paranoid if from time to time you treat yourself to a cream cake or bag of chips. Just don't make it a regular habit. Part of the joy of being a successful slimmer is the fact that you are in control and you have confidence in your ability to stay that way.

5 Continue to take regular aerobic exercise – 10–20 minutes, five times a week – as this is the most efficient way of burning fat off your body and maintaining your metabolic rate. Not only will it help you to stay fit and live longer, you will also be able to live your life more fully into the bargain.

6 Keeping those muscles in good shape is really important, so practise the toning workout two or three times a week. This will enable you to maintain your muscle tone and help counteract the body's natural inclination to lose muscle tissue as you get older. Remember, too, that regular exercise can help prevent the onset of osteoporosis.

7 Remember to maintain a good posture at all times of the day. Stand tall, pulling your tummy right in and your shoulders back and down, and try to add an inch to your height. A good posture is important if you want to keep your stomach flat, and it will help you to look younger too. The head is very heavy, weighing about 12 pounds – that's the weight of one of those great big ten-pin bowling balls. It is finely

balanced on top of your body, and if you get into bad posture habits you will be holding that heavy weight at the wrong angle. It stands to reason that if you adopt a good posture so that everything is in balance, your body will operate much more efficiently and stand you in good stead for years to come.

8   Keep a snugly fitting skirt or pair of trousers in your wardrobe to try on occasionally. This will form the most accurate gauge to your long-term progress in maintaining your new figure. As soon as the garment feels tighter, then step up on the exercise, cut back on the quantities of food you are eating and make doubly sure you are eating low fat. It's a whole lot easier to lose two pounds than it is to lose two stone.

9   Keep an eye on the scales. Weigh yourself once a week at the same time of day, wearing the same clothes or none at all. Make a note of your weight and if you find it creeping up, take the appropriate action.

10   Relax and enjoy your new-found figure. Don't become over-obsessive about your eating and exercise habits, but enjoy them and let them fit comfortably into your lifestyle. Don't become a diet bore but, instead, be an ambassador for healthy living.

# Dining out

Dining out is fun and there's no reason to forgo it in your new healthy eating regime. It is still possible to eat out and not gain loads of unwanted pounds. The key is not to feel guilty.

First, plan what you are going to wear. Choose something that will show off your new, slimmer figure. Any encouraging compliments will remind you of your success and prevent you from going overboard during the meal.

Start the evening with a long, slimline, non-alcoholic drink. This will help you to feel fuller more quickly.

Read the menu carefully and choose a light, low-calorie starter, perhaps melon with strawberries or other fruits. For your main course, avoid any food that is coated in pastry or breadcrumbs or that is served with butter or cream sauces. If in doubt ask the waiter for advice, explaining that you eat a low-fat diet for health reasons. Usually the staff will be only too pleased to assist, although don't let them try and convince you that extra virgin olive oil is low in fat! Don't forget to ask for your vegetables to be served without butter.

By all means, enjoy a glass of wine with your main course and top up with sparkling mineral water – drinking lots of mineral water will help to fill you up. For dessert, fresh strawberries or raspberries, oranges in liqueur, or pears in red wine, make an excellent choice. Instead of cream, ask for a small scoop of ice cream on top so that you don't feel deprived.

Finish with coffee or tea, but leave the mints and cheese and biscuits alone. Make sure you feel really full by the time you leave the table. Don't worry if you feel you have eaten too much – it doesn't do any harm to feel like that occasionally. The truth is, if you've been careful and followed the above advice, the next morning you'll find you probably haven't gained more than a few ounces. Just return to the diet, try to be a bit more active than usual and within a day or two any temporary damage will have been rectified.

*Bon appétit!*

# 10

## Success Stories

In this chapter I have included a selection of comments taken from the questionnaires and letters I received from both the trial dieters and those who followed the diet and exercise plan after publication of my original Flat Stomach Plan.

Susan Kristall of Leeds wrote:

'I feel much fitter and I am proud and thrilled because three out of the four weeks on the diet I have been on holiday in southern Spain and have not cheated once and have exercised daily. I am very proud of myself.'

Susan lost six and a half pounds during those four weeks and then continued on the diet. After eight weeks she had lost $13\frac{1}{2}$ pounds including five and a half inches off her abdomen and four and a half inches off her waist. She continued:

'I cannot believe my inch loss. It is incredible. I feel

fitter, very agile and supple and look so much younger, particularly in my face. It has made me feel on top of the world.'

Anne Marie MacLachlan from Inverness-shire lost a stone in four weeks. She wrote:

'I feel a new woman. I do not get so breathless when playing with my family or going up flights of stairs. I don't have to wait a couple of minutes before I speak.'

Pauline MacWhirter of Clydebank lost 10 pounds in four weeks and wrote:

'I suffer from stress and low self-esteem after personal problems and, although I have only been on the diet for four weeks, I can sense in myself a kind of confidence and achievement.'

Pauline continued on the diet for a further four weeks and lost a further four pounds, though she felt that she had lost more than this because family and neighbours had commented on the dramatic difference they could see. Pauline continued:

'Through losing weight and inches and receiving comments from family and friends, I have started to feel a lot better about myself and have even got the opportunity to return to work after being off for one and a half years.'

Zara Martin from London was a drama student in her early twenties when she went on the trial diet.

At 5ft 5in tall she weighed in at 12 stone. She had a typical dieting history, having tried various liquid meal replacements and had lost weight only to regain it again. After four weeks Zara had lost a stone and after four more weeks she had lost a further 12 pounds, making a total loss of 26 pounds. She lost four inches off her waist, three inches off her abdomen and five and a half inches off her hips.

Zara wrote:

'After eight weeks of following the diet and exercise regime I have so much more energy, feel fitter and am able to sustain exercise for a lot longer. I would recommend this diet to anyone who wants to lose weight, get fitter and healthier and eat sensibly. I feel I can say that this regime is for the rest of my life.'

Joanne Nutman from Dorset had been trying desperately to regain her figure after giving birth to her baby sixteen months previously when she applied to be part of the diet trial. Joanne lost seven pounds during the first four weeks and only four pounds during the next four, but she managed to lose four inches from her abdomen and three inches off her waist. She wrote:

'I had become so disillusioned after trying for so long to lose weight after having my daughter and nothing happening. After starting your diet and seeing its effects after just a month I feel so much better about myself. I am finding it such a novelty to keep trying on clothes from my wardrobe that I have not been able to get into for so long.'

After eight weeks Joanne wrote:

'I am thrilled with the results. I am amazed that by sticking to such straightforward guidelines, increasing my exercise and cutting out fat my weight has significantly reduced. It has made such a difference to my life.'

Patrician Pollard of Peterborough lost seven pounds in four weeks on the trial diet and four inches off her waist. She remarked:

'I have lost more inches than weight and that, for me, is the whole object. The diet is simplicity itself – so easy to follow.'

Patricia continued with the diet for another four weeks and lost a further three pounds plus lots more inches. She wrote:

'My general wellbeing is so great that my lust for living has jumped 100 per cent. Consequently my general health has benefited. Thank you, thank you, and thank you again. I never thought I would ever get slim again. The result is a new lease of life and the ability to cope again. My gratitude knows no bounds.'

Sarah Pulford from West Sussex tried everything from Weight Watchers to Slimfast. She had lost three and a half stone but had put it all back on again. At the beginning of the trial diet she weighed in at around 17 stone which was significantly overweight for her 5ft 7in height. After the first four weeks on the diet Sarah had lost 1st 2lb. After a further four weeks she had lost 2 stone and six inches off her abdomen and hips. She wrote on her questionnaire:

'Feeling lighter and fitter all round. I cannot believe how this diet has made a wonderful change to me.'

Sarah also reported that her back problem had eased tremendously and that clothes were beginning to fit better. Four months later Sarah wrote to me again:

'To date I have lost four stone and 36 inches – ten inches off my waist. I am so pleased to have taken part in your wonderful diet.'

Christine Ray from Devon lost nine pounds during the first four weeks of the diet and continued to lose thereafter. By the end of week eight she had lost five inches from her waist and abdomen and a total of 15 pounds. Christine, along with all the other trial dieters, were sworn to secrecy as to the source or purpose of the diet, so imagine my amusement when Christine wrote:

'I visited my GP recently. She said, "Good God, Christine, I'll have some of whatever it is you're on, you look great!" I laughed it off but she kept on at me. "Are you on a diet or something? You haven't looked this good in a long time." "Yes," I said, "but that is all I'm saying at the moment." We did laugh at the fact that if all her patients felt and looked as good as I did she would be out of a job!'

Shirley Royse from Cheshire was not greatly

overweight at 9st 7lb for her 5ft 1in height. But on her application form she wrote:

'I would like to be a new woman from head to toe.'

We included Shirley in the diet trial, despite the fact that she hadn't got too much weight to lose. After four weeks Shirley had lost seven pounds and several inches. Shirley continued on the diet and lost another four pounds during the next four weeks. She wrote:

'My skin is much better. The diet has given me much more energy and confidence. I look younger.'

After eight weeks she wrote:

'I think this diet is the only one that can start you on the way to healthy eating. I find for the first time in my 53 years I can eat sensibly and enjoy it.'

Christine Smith of Essex lost 1st 4lb in the first four weeks of the diet. She wrote:

'I am actually *enjoying* dieting. It has given me a feeling of wellbeing and I am *proud* of myself – something I have not felt for a very long time. The diet is easy to stick at and I now realise just how much fat I used to consume!'

Christine followed the diet for a further four weeks and lost a total of 24 pounds, including seven and a half inches from her abdomen. After eight weeks on the diet Christine wrote:

'I have been told by my husband and children that I

am a different person. I feel better about myself and I have been less moody. I shall continue on the diet in the hope of losing more weight. Whilst on my holiday I felt confident enough to wear my swimming costume (without a towel around me) and able to play in the swimming pool, jumping into my son's tyre and lilo without bursting them!'

Everyone who applied to join the trial diet had to send in a photograph of how they looked at that time. Sheila Smith from High Wycombe in Buckinghamshire also sent me an 'after' photograph which she had taken eight weeks after following the diet. She had lost ten pounds plus four inches off her abdomen and wrote:

'I feel more relaxed since finding a new hobby – walking! I had felt unwell since a back operation, taking no exercise, and constipation had been a problem. I have enjoyed the diet and it was lovely to still be able to have the occasional low-fat ice cream. The best thing is I have got rid of my tummy and brought out my straight skirts again. Hooray!'

The difference between Sheila's 'before' and 'after' photographs was dramatic even though she had only lost 10 pounds. From the photographs it looked as if she had lost two stone.

Tina Wright from Wiltshire lost seven pounds in the first four weeks on the diet and a further eight pounds in the following four. Tina wrote:

'Thank you from the bottom of my heart for including me as part of your trial team. I feel and look fantastic and will continue in the same vein. I feel fitter and have more energy. I can chase my children without so much of the wobble and blimp-like feeling. My skin is certainly clearer and my posture has improved. This diet is marvellous, very simple to follow and stick to even with a husband and four children to include.'

After publication of my original Flat Stomach Plan I began to receive further letters. Denise Warren reported that she had lost 12 pounds and 21 inches overall in the first four weeks. Her letter read:

'I feel I must write to say how thrilled I was with your Flat Stomach Plan. I shall recommend it to everyone. I'm 50 years old and I have always maintained a weight of between 9st 10lbs and just over 10 stone, then I realised my clothes were getting tighter. I weighed in at 10st 7lb and my stomach spoilt all my clothes as it stuck out. I have slimmed before but *never* stuck to an exercise plan. I used to say I haven't got time for all that and it isn't necessary, but you have proved me wrong. It's fantastic. I never expected to lose all those inches – $16\frac{1}{2}$ in total and I feel great. My dresses look a lot better – it's a marvellous plan and I feel like shouting from the roof tops.'

Every day of the week I receive a vast mail bag which is carefully sorted by my wonderful office staff. When we receive a letter such as the one below from Rose Valentine from Hertfordshire it reminds us all of the enormous help that the diet and exercises give to those who follow them. This is Rose's letter:

'I feel fabulous! I have just completed four weeks of the Flat Stomach Plan; I feel better than I have done for a very long time and I have lost seven pounds without feeling continuously starving hungry! It's been brilliant. The meals are tasty and interesting – I can eat heaps and heaps – and the exercises have made a vast improvement to my shape. On Saturday I spent half an hour trying on clothes that haven't fitted me for ages and they are all really loose now.

'And that to my mind is the crux of the matter. On other diets I have felt hungry and seen or felt no real difference and therefore given up. With this diet, I, who have a huge appetite, can eat so much that I don't get hungry, and the exercises spurred me on to do greater things. I now go to two aerobics classes of one hour each every week. Even although I ride horses very regularly and considered myself to be quite fit to begin with (ha ha) this diet and exercise plan has shown me that I was wrong. But now I feel so much better and, because I can see and feel results, it encourages me to carry on.

'This year I will be 40 and I didn't want to wake up on my birthday being flabby, fat and 40, and now thanks to you I won't be. Thank you so much for that! Just one point – I measured myself at the beginning of the first week but when I went to measure myself the following week I felt that I wasn't measuring the same place as before, if you get my gist! After that I didn't measure myself at all but as I can see the results I don't think it matters!'

There's much concern these days about young girls dieting excessively. On the one hand, some are aiming for ridiculously thin and unnatural bodies, while others suffer from overweight which is ruining their young lives. My view is that young people should be more active and should eat for health without getting bogged down with calorie counting. Having said that I was delighted to receive the following letter from Louise Charles from Lancashire. Louise is 16 years old and 5ft 6½in tall. When she started on the Flat Stomach Plan diet she was between 2 and 3 stone overweight.

'After years of constant dieting and the depression that goes with it, I had finally had enough. I noticed that you had a new diet plan out. I knew your diets worked after following the Hip and Thigh diet. That gave amazing results but in the end it was my willpower that gave in. So on New Year's day, I started the Flat Stomach Plan and weighed in at my heaviest weight ever – 14 stone. For a 16 year old, that was a bit too heavy. One month later, I am 11 pounds lighter and 14 inches less. Of course I have a few stone to go but I am a much happier person. On day 24 it was my 17th birthday. I started my driving lessons and felt so confident about them. (Confidence is something I have always lacked and this has got on many people's nerves.) The previous weekend I had the confidence to celebrate my birthday by going to a club with my friend and finding I had the stamina to dance for three and a half hours non-stop. I have so much more energy already, I can't wait until I have lost all my weight!'

Mrs J N from East Yorkshire bought a copy of the Flat Stomach Plan since she wanted to lose three stone. She filled in the questionnaire in the book. Her age range is between 65 and 74, her height is 5ft 4in and her commencing weight was 12st 7lb. Mrs J N wrote:

'The reason for the alterations on the questionnaire is that I was losing weight and inches so quickly, so I left it for a few more weeks before I posted it to you. The total loss in weight is from 12½ stone to 9st 4lb to date, plus all those inches. It is possible if you are determined to do it. Thank you. I have wanted to go back to my normal weight for years.'

Mrs J N had lost six inches from her waist, five inches from her abdomen and seven inches off her hips. She went on to add on the questionnaire that her angina, her heart and eye problems had all improved.

Mrs Beck of the West Midlands followed the diet and exercises in the book for four weeks and lost ten pounds. She also lost five inches from around her abdomen and three inches off her waist. She sent an accompanying letter with her completed questionnaire:

'I watched you and your dieters on *This Morning* and I was so encouraged that I decided to send for the book. I am so glad that I did. My husband also joined me on the diet and it was so much easier cooking meals for the two of us. The food was delicious and we are carrying on until I reach my ideal weight. I never thought I would want to carry on when I started the diet, but you don't feel as if you are missing out. I definitely feel more energetic, but the best thing of all is that people I see on a regular basis comment on how slim I look, even though I still have got quite a way to go. So I want to thank you very much for helping me achieve something I didn't think I could do.'

Valerie Aston from Hampshire wrote:

'I am so pleased I saw your book and I have already recommended it to friends. I was only 1st 2lb overweight but, even so, I was having breathing problems and felt like a landed whale as all the weight seemed to be around my stomach. I needed trousers two sizes bigger than the rest of me. As I am only 4ft 10in tall, 8st 2lb was a lot for me to carry around. In only four weeks I have lost four inches from the stomach area and four pounds in weight, and that without the exercises. I have a lot of very bad tension headaches and found that the exercises gave me a headache (through getting out of breath). I hope, as I slim down, to try them again. In place of them I am walking much more. I walk to town, shop, then come home on the bus – in all I am walking continuously for two or three hours which I don't find difficult at all. I also cycle more often, around the common where I live, and in the summer I hope to go swimming more often.

'Middle age crept up on me unawares (I'm 42). I suppose I assumed I would stay at 7st for ever. I think the positive thoughts at the end of each day are excellent – very encouraging. I feel so much better now and I love the recipes. I haven't tried them all as some foods don't agree with me, but apart from that they are so tasty and filling.'

June Longton from Lancashire wrote:

'I really loved this diet. I must admit I was a little disappointed at first. I only lost two pounds in my first week, but then I measured myself and was surprised at the inches I had lost. I followed the diet for four weeks and lost 18 inches. I was so thrilled. Then there was the food. I just didn't feel like I was on a diet – the recipes were delicious. What I liked most was that it was all real food, not frozen or pre-made.

'My husband followed the diet with me. He lost more weight than me but the same number of inches. I am going to continue on the diet until I get to nine stone. I am 5ft 4in but I am staying with the low fat – it's a new way of life. I must say as a chocoholic – or rather ex-chocoholic – I haven't cheated once, and because of the dessert recipes, I haven't missed chocolate at all. Thank you for a lovely diet.'

I received this letter from Marie Mahony in Queensland, Australia:

'Thank you for your wonderful Flat Stomach Plan book. I found it in the local newsagent one weekend when I was feeling very depressed about my body shape and my lack of self-discipline. I feel like a new person! I have lost four kilos but I feel so much trimmer and fitter. Your diet plan has been a little difficult for me to follow – some foods are not available here. However I have tried to follow a very basic, fat-free diet. The daily exercise plan has been wonderful – just what I needed. Thank you again. Probably most of all, I loved your positive thoughts each day.'

Angela Langley was mentioned earlier in the book. Angela wrote:

'I hope you don't mind me using your Christian name but after working out to your Flat Stomach Plan video since the middle of January this year I now feel that you are part of the family.

'I would like to start by saying that on 17 January I weighed in on my scales at home at 14st 10lb and with my height being 5ft 7in I was quite a lot heavier than I should have been. I had decided that I would try to lose four stone and then if I was successful I would try to fine-tune down to a weight that I thought I would be happy with. I converted the four stone to pounds and after watching you on one of the *This Morning* programmes made a graph with weeks at the bottom and pounds at the side. I decided to work backwards from 56 pounds with a stone on each page, so in all I had four pages.

'I also purchased the Flat Stomach Plan book and measured myself towards the end of January. I have been weighing in every week on Sundays and measuring myself every two weeks. I was completely amazed at how quickly my weight and measurements changed. I am now into my 25th week and I have lost an unbelievable 4st 7lb. My bust measurement has gone down by seven and a half inches, waist by nine inches, widest part by nine inches and hips by ten inches. I felt I had to write to tell you how much you have changed my life in such a short time. I have so much energy and feel a lot more confident just walking down the street. I have recently bought a bike and enjoy riding out with the children. The only thing left for me to do is to lose my last 8lb and go out shopping for a new set of clothes.'

Sheila Cargius of Clwyd lost a stone in four weeks on the trial and wrote:

'I feel so much healthier after just four weeks. I find I am eating much healthier food and more importantly eating properly – there are no faddy foods or regimes – it is just sensible choices. Everybody comments not only on my weight loss but how much better I look and I certainly feel so. I have so much more energy, my nails have grown for the first time in ages and it is really spurring me on.'

Johanna Castles from Worcestershire lost 16 pounds

in the first four weeks of the trial and had lost 27 pounds after eight weeks. She wrote:

'I feel marvellous! My cellulite has almost all gone. My husband has lost a stone over the eight weeks, although he has not consciously dieted. It has made us both very aware of our diets. The eating programme has saved us money.'

Hazel Thomas from Wolverhampton wrote:

'At the end of 1994 I took part in the *This Morning* new trial diet which has since become the Flat Stomach Plan. During the trial I lost nine pounds and 24 inches and since then I have continued with the diet. I would like to thank you for the Flat Stomach Plan as to date I have lost 1st 8lb and 32.4 inches. I intend to continue with the diet as it has made me feel amazing.'

Anthony Edwards was one of our male trial dieters. Anthony, who lives in Manchester, lost 1st 4lb in the first four weeks and wrote:

'Since starting this diet I have more energy, and I can walk without getting out of breath. My sleeping has also improved since starting the diet.'

He also went on to say that he was not as bad tempered as before, that he felt more confident, and looked significantly slimmer. Anthony continued:

'This diet is one of the finest things I have ever done.'

After eight weeks Anthony had lost a magnificent 29 pounds. He wrote:

'I am now fitter than I was 20 years ago (as a police officer). I do thirty minutes exercise every day. I do not get breathless any more. I would like to thank everyone involved in getting this diet going. The benefit to me personally has been fantastic. I have been more pleasant to live with (so my wife says).'

Losing weight and getting into shape is never straightforward. I hope that these letters and quotes from various questionnaires will serve to inspire you when you need it. I hope you will never tire of reading them.

# 11

## The Benefits to Health

Apart from the obvious changes to the way they looked and felt when they lost weight and inches, many followers of the Flat Stomach Plan also experienced significant benefits to their health too.

In this chapter I have included a selection of their comments and grouped them under specific headings for easy reference.

I would add that, while many people enjoyed dramatic improvements to their health and general wellbeing, this chapter in no way is suggesting that everyone will benefit in the same way. In any event, if you have any medical condition, it is always advisable to consult your doctor first before embarking on any diet or fitness programme.

### Arthritis

Patricia Lewins from West Yorkshire wrote:

'I suffer from arthritis and a back injury but after

only a few weeks I noticed the difference. My joints were not as painful. In fact, the difference is amazing.'

Ann Erwin from Merseyside lost 12 pounds in the first four weeks on the diet and then continued to lose a further nine pounds by week eight. She lost a remarkable six inches off her waist and five inches off her abdomen and wrote:

'As I suffer from arthritis of the spine I am now more agile and it is great to be able to get out of a chair without having to be heaved out. Also I found that my night sweats have subsided.'

Mrs Brenda Mallett from Surrey lost 13 pounds in eight weeks and wrote that she was now more energetic, less tired and since losing weight had reduced the pain in her hips caused by arthritis. Her hot flushes had also gone since starting the diet. She went on to say:

'This is the best diet I have tried. I would certainly recommend it to anyone who hates dieting because this is not like being on a diet.'

Dori Piper from East Sussex lost 18 pounds in eight weeks and explained that she used to have very bad early morning catarrhal headaches and nausea, but they had now completely cleared. Her arthritic pain is now minimal and the cellulite on her legs has reduced. She explained that her general sense of wellbeing and energy was much improved. And went on to say:

'Perhaps the most important benefit for me has been the dramatic change in eating habits. No more embarrassing rumbling tummy, no more sick, hungry feeling and then a binge! I still can't believe I can eat ice cream, marmalade, meringue! Every previous diet I have done (and there were many) was a crash diet and always a flop.'

Mrs J A from South Yorkshire wrote:

'Firstly a very big thank you for your diet. As you can see from my questionnaire I am very overweight and always have been for as long as I can remember. I have been on this-diet and that-diet and have always lost interest. You have also saved me from the ghastly task of having my stomach stapled to aid my weight loss. I began your plan on 3 January and an appointment came for me to go in on 15 January. I had been put on the waiting list two or three years ago, weighing 17st 12lb. My weight then ballooned to over 20 stone – I don't know how much over as my scales only go up to 19 stone! I then thought about my two children aged four and five and the fact that my father's side of the family died at around 60 through heart attacks and (funny though it is) how much my husband would have to spend on a coffin, and if I died upstairs how would they get me down? That is when I began my calorie counting. This was June 1994 and up to Christmas I got down to about 18st 10lb. Then, whilst munching a jam sandwich and a cup of tea, I read about your Flat Stomach Plan and decided to give it a try. "Just another diet, more calorie counting" went through my mind. On January 3 I started the diet revolution. It is fantastic! I went into town the following day to get the workout video. When I began I could only do the toning exercises and level 1 aerobics. Now I can happily do the toning, level 2 aerobics, and I also exercise to my other new video (*Rosemary Conley All New Hip and Thigh Workout*). I do these shortly after my husband goes to work at 6am and I feel I have achieved so much that it sets me up for the day. Apart from my increased fitness levels, although I still look like an egg on legs – but a slimmer egg of course – I have bags more confidence and the sense of feeling that I will get down to the 13 stone I was when I got married eight years ago, hopefully by October (my wedding anniversary) but if not then, Christmas. Then it will be 9st 9lb about the average I think for my height.

'My health has improved too. I have arthritis in both of my knees and for ever swollen ankles. They stopped me getting about easily in the morning but, thanks to you, I feel like a new person. My husband also follows the plan and I am sure he enjoys the meals too. I have suffered from back pain for a number of years and the only advice I got from my GP was "lose weight". Now I have and I can feel the difference.

'I can't wait to discover what life holds for me when I reach my 13 stone target weight, but it is amazing that I have only just started to wear more fashionable clothes for my age (I am 26) instead of the manufacturers' frump stuff they automatically think fat people want to wear. I know I have a long way to go but I am sure with your plan on my side I'll get there.'

Elizabeth Craig lost 10 pounds during the first four weeks on the diet and another eight pounds in the second four. She also lost six inches from her waist and four and a half inches from her abdomen. After four weeks she wrote on her questionnaire:

'I have stopped taking my drugs for arthritis. I have found myself running up stairs (first time for years). My GP, who is also a friend, is pleased with how well I look.

'It's the first diet I have lost weight without looking haggard. As a bell ringer I now have to wear a belt to hold my trousers up. I lunch every day with a retired doctor who is very impressed with the balanced meals I have. Thank you for my new life.'

NB Any reduction in medication should only be done under medical supervision.

## Asthma and Breathing Problems

Elaine Swaincot of Derbyshire wrote:

'Since I started to lose weight I am less breathless than I have been for a long time and I am far more energetic and mobile – it's fabulous!'

Elaine lost 13 pounds in the first four weeks and then continued on the diet and filled in a second questionnaire after eight weeks by which time she had lost a further seven pounds and five inches from her waist, abdomen, hips and widest part. After eight weeks she wrote:

'The continued weight loss, although slower now, has made it easier to get about and I have been less asthmatic than normal which has given me a feeling of much better general wellbeing. Fabulous! I have never found a diet so interesting – having the hard work taken out of it. It has been super.'

Patricia O'Neal from Bury lost a stone in four weeks and after a further four weeks her total weight loss was 24 pounds. She wrote:

'I am asthmatic and used to become breathless on exertion. Having lost weight I can now run upstairs without my inhaler. I work on an elderly care ward. It was so rewarding to have my clients commenting on my weight loss.'

Joyce Neal from Essex had previously suffered with her breathing and had been for tests for asthma. After four weeks on the diet Joyce had lost 13 pounds and wrote:

'I cannot get over how my breathing is so much better. I have been doing one to two miles running when I can and on Wednesdays and Fridays I run with a group that runs for charity. I ran four miles non-stop. It took me 50 minutes but because my breathing allowed me to, I did not stop once and I feel great. I have never run four miles in my life before, and to think I am still overweight. What I will be able to achieve later!'

Lynn Campbell from Tyne and Wear wrote:

'I don't get so out of breath and, believe it or not, my hot flushes have almost stopped! I also feel better about myself and I can run upstairs without panting. The first week I lost five pounds. I feel great. After three weeks I stopped thinking of myself as on a diet. I feel as though I am eating properly and sensibly. It is healthy eating and I am enjoying it.'

Lynn lost nine pounds in the first four weeks and continued on the diet and lost 13 pounds in eight weeks. She then wrote:

'My breathing is great, I can run upstairs and my hot flushes have almost gone. My confidence and morale have been given a big boost. I am standing tall – not slouching. My friend said even my eyes are brighter. I know I will continue on this great eating plan and get to my target weight. I can't thank you enough. My husband is delighted with the new me. Every time I sat down to dinner, he would say, "Are you sure you can have *all* of that?" I ate more than he did! Both myself and my doctor are delighted.'

Jane Calvert of Derbyshire lost 14 pounds in the first four weeks and a further seven pounds in the following four. She wrote:

'My asthma seems to have improved, I certainly don't get as breathless and I am definitely a lot fitter. My back and neck problems are also greatly improved.'

Maureen Brookes lost 1st 1lb in four weeks and wrote:

'This diet has stopped me being breathless, and I don't feel as tired.'

It is obvious that if once we lose weight the body does not have to work so hard to move around. When we feel physical benefits such as not being out of breath, this encourages us to stick with the diet so that we don't regain the weight. Life is so much easier if we are our 'normal' weight and are not carrying around that spare 'suitcase' with us everywhere we go.

## Backache

Jane Ahmad from Hampshire lost seven pounds during the first four weeks and six pounds during the second four weeks and reduced her weight to 9st 5lb. On her questionnaire she stated that she had no more backache and that her self-esteem had returned and this had lifted her depression. She told me that she was able to move more freely and was more supple now and she added: 'My children have almost stopped calling me Mrs Blobby!' She went on to say that she could now run and catch the children and was able to enjoy her dancing now that she is not carrying so much weight around with her.

Janice Garratt from Essex lost 17 pounds in eight weeks and wrote:

'I had lower back problems before starting the diet but now I can honestly say I cannot remember the last time I had lower back ache. I am so pleased with this diet. I have never been able to lose so much so quickly *and* eat so much. It has definitely opened my eyes to how many biscuits I was eating before. I will definitely continue with the diet to lose the rest of my weight. I can't thank you enough.'

Susan Jamieson from Stockton on Tees lost 14 pounds in eight weeks and wrote:

'My backache has gone, my breast pain has gone, I just feel so much better, more positive and much more energetic. I have really enjoyed the past eight weeks on this diet and exercise plan, so much so that I am keeping on with it until all my excess fat has gone. Before, exercise to me was a dirty word, but now I go to exercise classes twice a week and I have bought a second-hand bike.'

Hazel Thomas from the West Midlands lost 1st 2lb in eight weeks and wrote:

'My back has become almost pain free after years of pain and extensive medical treatment. I find your combined diet and fitness plan has given me an energy boost and I have thus been able to reduce my weight and shake into gear muscles that have been dormant for years. I have joined a gym and find the encouragement of fellow members a great motiv-ation. I have even begun to notice an improvement in my knees which are arthritic and have previously caused great discomfort. I intend to continue on this plan as it has really changed my life and my whole outlook.'

Hazel went on to say:

'I took a fortnight's holiday during the trial and amazed my husband by sticking to the plan. He was astonished when he discovered just how wide a choice the diet offered. He sat in restaurants saying, "I don't think you should be having that." I proved my point when I returned home four pounds lighter. He is so impressed he wants to join the trial!'

Sue Pearce from Surrey asked to be given the Flat Stomach Plan book as a Christmas present. She started the diet on 2 January and in four weeks lost a stone. She wrote:

'Our cupboards hold completely different foods now. The first week we found it a bit tough but we soon got into it. After four weeks we are delighted but won't stop here. I was getting a lot of backache and bust pain. The pains have gone and the exercises help my back.'

Mrs P from London lost 14 pounds in four weeks and wrote:

'The exercises have really improved my posture. I have had a troublesome back problem for years and the back-strengthening exercises have really improved that. Also the great feeling of getting into my clothes without having to wrestle to do up buttons and zips. I have been a widow for almost seven years and two years ago I met a widower and we are getting married on 1 July. It makes me feel great to know I will look so much better in my wedding outfit.'

NB Anyone who has a back problem should obviously consult with their doctor before taking any form of exercise.

## Diabetes

Because my diet is high in carbohydrates it is particularly well suited to diabetics. Meals can be broken up for anyone suffering from this condition in order that the necessary carbohydrate can be eaten at the appropriate times. Providing the quantities are not exceeded, weight loss will still be enjoyed.

Diane Griffiths of Northampton lost 13 pounds in the first four weeks of the diet and wrote:

'I can't believe it was so easy. I hope to continue to do as well in the next four weeks. It was easier than I ever expected any diet to be.'

Diane continued with the diet and lost a further nine pounds in the following four weeks and wrote:

'It was so easy to incorporate my diabetic diet into the trial. It is the best diet for diabetics I have ever found. I have got back into my jeans that I haven't worn for over two years. I hope to continue until I get to my goal weight. Thank you for giving me my confidence and my figure back. I hope you are as impressed with the result of the trial as I am.'

## Eczema

Sue Hughes of Liverpool followed the diet for four weeks and lost 15 pounds. Sue wrote:

'I have eczema on my eyelids. Since being on the diet this has improved greatly.'

Lyn Fletcher from Scotland lost 12 pounds in four weeks on the diet and wrote:

'I suffer with eczema and have seen a marked improvement in the condition of my skin.'

## Headaches

Pauline Smith from Weston-super-Mare lost seven pounds in the first four weeks on the trial diet and wrote:

'I suffer with a lot of headaches, cluster headaches, migraines and stress-related headaches, but during the last two weeks I haven't had a headache! I feel more relaxed. I don't know if that's because I am losing weight and I am pleased or because of some of the foods I have cut out.'

Mrs L M from Ipswich bought a copy of the Flat

Stomach Plan and lost eight pounds in her first four weeks of following the diet. She filled in the questionnaire at the back of the book and accompanied it with the following letter:

'I am writing to thank you for showing some new eating habits to one self-confessed chocoholic.

'I intended to follow the plan for only four very strict weeks. In that time I not only lost weight but also began to feel a lot younger and healthier. Stress was reduced and headaches are practically non-existent. After the four weeks were up I went back to my old eating habits for a weekend and I felt an absolute wreck. So, although I am fairly happy now with my weight, I shall still follow the plan purely for the health benefits that I am enjoying.'

Jean Skelton from Shropshire volunteered to be part of our trial team. Jean is an attractive 42-year-old who attends a local Rosemary Conley Diet & Fitness Club. Jean had plenty of weight to lose but enjoyed the astonishing benefits of losing 26 pounds in the first four weeks. The fact that Jean was part of a trial team had inspired her to follow the diet strictly. She wrote:

'After following this diet to the letter I felt happier and healthier whilst I was losing weight. In fact, this diet has shown I can lose weight, hopefully on a permanent basis – something that has eluded me so far. I find that I can do more things more easily, I also find my staff can get past me better in our very narrow kitchen here at the Swan at Foreton.'

Jean continued on the diet for a further four weeks and lost a total of 44 pounds in eight weeks. This was an astonishing achievement. Along with the weight she lost six inches off her bust, seven inches off her waist, six inches off her abdomen, nine inches off her hips and six inches off her widest part. Jean wrote:

'Since I have lost so much weight a previously difficult hernia operation will now be possible. I can also beat the dog in a race up the stairs!'

## Heart Problems

Mrs Catherine Davies lives in Ross-shire in northern Scotland. When Catherine commenced the trial she weighed 10st 2lb which was heavy for her 5ft 2in frame. Catherine lost 13 pounds during the first four weeks on the diet and a total of 21 pounds after eight weeks to reach her target weight.

'I suffer from chronic heart disease, hence the reason for not being able to do the exercises. But now I find I do not get so breathless and find I can walk a lot more easily. I am sticking to your diet and love it.'

Beryl Bull from Kent had undergone heart surgery but had been told by her specialist that she should do some light exercise. Beryl was selected to be part of the trial team. In the first four weeks Beryl lost 12 pounds and wrote:

'I feel much fitter and happier. Also I had a blood

cholesterol test after only two weeks on the diet and it came down to 5.7. That has made everything even better. I know it has only been four weeks but I have lost a total of 12 pounds and nine inches. I don't feel so lethargic. I am never hungry, so I don't want to nibble in between meals. I feel confident that this diet is going to help me far more than others have in the past. I plan to eat this diet for a healthy lifetime.'

Jeannette Bland from north Yorkshire also suffers with a heart condition. Despite being told by the doctor to keep her weight down she found her willpower was zero, so she was anxious to be part of the trial team. After four weeks, Jeannette had lost 17 pounds. She wrote:

'Because of the weight loss I feel far more energetic and not so sluggish and tired when I am at work or out walking. The diet made me actually *think* about what I was eating, and I realise that I hadn't been having enough fruit and vegetables but far too much fatty food. I also realised how much I pick when I am preparing a meal – a low-fat diet can only improve my health because having a heart complaint, I am always being told to eat a healthy diet.'

Jeannette continued on the diet for a further four weeks and lost a total of 26 pounds. She wrote:

'My doctor is very pleased because of my heart condition. My own feelings can be said with one comment – Yippee!

'I walk my dog every morning but since I have

started the diet, what used to be a stroll has turned into a fast walk for my 15-minute exercise period. One particular morning, I suddenly became aware that the dog wasn't with me and when I looked around, she was lying in the middle of the road about 200 yards behind me with a look on her face that said, "You must be joking." She has also taken to rolling over on her back with her feet in the air when I do the exercises!'

Mrs Ann Leonard from Cumbria lost 13 pounds in the first four weeks on the diet. She wrote:

'I don't feel as sluggish. The girls at work commented that I was getting back to my sprightly, bubbly self. I have stopped getting palpitations when climbing the stairs and I am not as tired and weary as I have been lately. My health was suffering because of my weight problem. Now I have lost nearly a stone I seem to have a lot more energy through exercising and eating more healthily. My knees don't ache as much as they did at work. I am no longer consti-pated, my shoes fit better and my rings are no longer tight.'

## Hiatus Hernia and Digestive Problems

Ann Zinkel lives in Edinburgh. In the first four weeks of following the diet Ann lost 10lb and wrote:

'I feel a lot fitter. I can walk further distances, my tummy muscles keep pulling me in, reminding me to walk straighter instead of waddling! Your simple but effective exercises are a pleasure to do. I really look forward to doing them. My doctor, who I have been registered with for 26 years, is very pleased. He says your diet is doing more for my tummy (hiatus hernia) than he has ever been able to do.'

Ann continued on the diet and lost a total of 14 pounds after eight weeks. She wrote:

'Eight weeks ago I would not have thought it possible that I would reach this weight. It gives me even more determination to reach my target.'

Mrs V W from Cheshire lost ten pounds in the first four weeks plus seven and a half inches off her waist. She wrote:

'My back trouble has improved considerably. I have suffered from stomach ulcers, and I have had no digestive problems since starting the diet. This diet has been a real life-saver for me. I had become very low, my health was not good at all due to being overweight and being extremely unfit. Now I have so much more energy and an increased feeling of wellbeing. I look and feel so much better.'

By week eight Mrs V W had lost 20 pounds. She had lost nine inches from her waist and five inches from her abdomen. She wrote:

'My back trouble has improved dramatically. I have not had any problems with my stomach (i.e. ulcers) whilst being on the diet – hurray I feel great! The diet has changed my life. I had a terrible problem with food (compulsive eating). I almost was going to go to a clinic for eating disorders! I chose to follow the trial, thank goodness! The bingeing is over, I feel great, I can run!! I have joined a health club and take regular classes.'

Mrs T C from Middlesex lost seven pounds in the first four weeks and wrote:

'I have a hiatus hernia, and the pain and discomfort I suffered, particularly at night, have completely gone. I feel more lively and energetic. I have given my husband the same meals, more or less. He is recovering well from a recent heart attack, and the diet plan has helped him to reduce weight too. We are very pleased with the results so far though I do wish the weight loss was greater!'

Helen Alexander from Fife lost 13 pounds in the first four weeks together with five inches off her waist and 3in off her abdomen. Helen wrote:

'I feel much fitter, have easier movement, no bloated feeling, no indigestion and the sense of wellbeing that comes from doing something about my weight problem.'

After a further four weeks, Helen's total weight loss came to 20 pounds. She also lost six inches from her waist and five inches from her abdomen. She wrote:

'I feel much fitter, stronger in my legs – it's easier to

go up hills without puffing. I have no heartburn or indigestion. I can now get into a skirt that I haven't been able to wear. I've forgotten what a biscuit tastes like never mind a chocolate one!'

Rita Bennett from Buckinghamshire lost 13 pounds in the first four weeks on the diet and a further three pounds by week eight. The interesting fact was that after four weeks Rita lost only one inch from her waist and abdomen, but by week eight she had lost two and a half inches from her waist and five inches from her abdomen. She wrote:

'My hiatus hernia no longer gives me problems. I am also sleeping better.'

Janet Bradley from Devon lost seven pounds during the first four weeks on the diet and a further five pounds by week eight. She lost four inches from her abdomen. After four weeks Janet wrote:

'I am less breathless when walking up the stairs and up hills. Before joining one of your diet and fitness classes I suffered a lot with a hiatus hernia – since that day these problems reduced drastically and since being on this trial diet I have had no problems at all. I have found that my weight loss occurred in weeks one and three and no loss in weeks two and four.'

After eight weeks Janet wrote:

'I have had no problems at all with my hiatus hernia which previously caused me a lot of trouble. I have also had far fewer headaches.'

## High Blood Pressure

Kay White of Essex lost eight pounds in four weeks. She lost a further four pounds by week eight and a remarkable five inches off her abdomen. Kay wrote:

'I had high blood pressure but because I have lost weight, when I visited the consultant my blood pressure was normal. Although I have a bad back, the exercises do me good. I feel healthier and younger. I don't feel I am on a diet and I don't call it that. I call it eating clean, healthy food.'

Rosemary Barnett from Surrey is a retired district nurse. After four weeks on the diet Rosemary had lost ten pounds and by week eight she had lost 16 pounds plus six inches from her waist and three inches from her abdomen. She wrote:

'My aches and pains are not as evident as they were. I can walk without getting out of breath. I genuinely feel a difference. I have more movement and much less fatigue. The best surprise was my blood pressure recording at the doctors – 130 over 80. It has not registered as normal as this in the last five years. My usual recordings have been 160 over 100. This is a real bonus. I almost sent my doctor's blood pressure up with surprise!'

Betty Arbuckle from Lancashire lost 16 pounds during the first four weeks of the diet and a total of 23lb after eight weeks. She lost eight inches off her waist and seven inches off her abdomen. Betty wrote:

'I just had to write to let you know how thrilled and delighted my doctor was when I went to the surgery for a six-month blood pressure and medication review. My doctor had requested that I should lose some weight 12 months ago but I never could. I hadn't told her that I had been picked for your trial diet. She was delighted with the amount of weight I had lost. In fact, I have been taken off the water tablets I took daily and I am now only on the blood pressure tablets. Hopefully in two months, when I next go to see her, I may have that strength reduced. Being a nurse, I should have lost weight sooner, but thanks to the trial diet I have now done it, and feel so much healthier and fitter.'

Angela Townsend from Buckinghamshire lost 19 pounds during the first four weeks on the diet and a total of 23 pounds after eight weeks. She lost four inches from her waist and five inches from her abdomen. She wrote:

'My blood pressure has reduced, causing far less headaches. Having been on the trial for four weeks I feel so much better and energetic, and because I can see the weight loss taking place it gives me the willpower to carry on with the diet. People at work are really commenting on how well I look and are giving me all the support I need to make it work.'

After the eighth week Angela wrote:

'My blood pressure is coming down to a normal level. I have now got so much more energy and "get-up-

and-go" that my husband can't keep up with me! I have far fewer headaches. I can honestly say I have never felt so fit and healthy and I am going to stay like this for ever.'

## High Cholesterol

When Mrs N R from Cheshire applied to participate in the trial diet she explained that she had high blood pressure and high cholesterol for which she received medication. After four weeks, Mrs N R wrote:

'The good news is that my cholesterol, which was 8.2 before starting your diet, has now gone down to 7.0. I am very pleased about this.'

After eight weeks, Mrs N R wrote:

'Both my blood pressure and cholesterol level have decreased.'

## Irritable Bowel Syndrome

Michelle Barkley from Cleveland lost 12 pounds during the first four weeks and a further eight pounds during the second four weeks. By week eight she had lost six and a half inches from her waist and seven inches from her abdomen. Michelle wrote:

'I have been dieting on and off since the age of ten, and I have tried almost every diet available. At 23 this diet feels like a gift because the weight and inches are coming off in the areas where I am biggest and from the places I have wanted to reduce for years. I am very pleased to be part of the trial team and my health is quite different because I feel I am full of energy.

'In the past couple of years I have occasionally suffered from irritable bowel syndrome but I have not suffered at all on your wonderful diet plan. I am determined to continue this diet because of the improvement in my shape. I have gained confidence because I feel better in having a new figure. I feel like a different person and have had a great boost in my self-confidence. Even friends and family have noticed.'

Joan Badbrick from Durham lost 11 pounds in four weeks on the trial diet. She wrote:

'I suffer from irritable bowel syndrome and had lots of pain in my stomach before this diet.'

## ME

Shirley McGee from Northern Ireland applied to be part of the trial diet. This is what she wrote on her application form:

'I had a bout of ME in 1985 which left me unfit to cope with the heavy workload of teaching English full time to A-level students. Because I need the organisation and support of committing myself to a scheme outside of my home, my retired husband has taken over the kitchen, the cooking and shopping and now meals and treats are almost non-stop. The menu is olive oil with everything and it tastes great. Save me!'

Shirley followed the diet for the first four weeks and lost six pounds. She wrote:

'Since following the trial diet I feel much less tired and have greater clarity of thought and improved concentration, so much so that I have been able to drive to nearby towns for leisurely shopping without the impatient husband/driver and inevitable time limit. I am delighted to have lost weight and inches despite the fact that I can only exercise with moderation due a long-term ME condition. My spine feels straight and my posture has improved.'

Shirley continued with the diet for a further four weeks and lost a total of ten pounds, plus four inches from her abdomen and two and a half inches from her waist. She wrote:

'This trial diet has given me new hope. I look better, feel better, I can think more clearly and I am able to drive again. Now I know I can keep my shape under control without damaging my health by starving and bingeing and with long-term ME good nourishing food is vital.

'Because of ME I have to be sensible about not overdoing exercise and so I just increased my walking little by little and did the toning exercises for only a few repetitions to begin with, building to a modest level slowly (sudden or undue exertions can increase the ME symptoms of pain and loss of strength in the muscles and joints). I am very very excited with what your plan has helped me achieve and I am going to stay with it. My spine is straight and stronger, my shape is trim, my spirits have lifted and life seems good.'

## Multiple Sclerosis

Susan O'Connor from East Sussex bought a copy of the Flat Stomach Plan and followed it very strictly. Susan wrote to me, enclosing her completed questionnaire:

'I have followed your plan since you first came on TV this year, even though I am in a wheelchair with MS. You will see my weight loss and inch loss is fantastic. I can't even stand so my husband helped me to do the exercises on the bed. I am delighted, so is he. He says I am much easier to lift now. I intend to carry on with it for a while as I would like to get down to 9st 3lb and firm up a little more.'

Susan lost a total of 3st 10lb and her inch loss was quite outstanding. She lost three inches off her bust, 11 inches off her waist, 15½ inches from her abdomen, ten from her hips, 15 from her widest part, eight inches off each thigh and four and a half inches from above each knee. Her figure is now a trim 36–27–37 which, for her 5ft 8in height is fantastic.

This letter and completed questionnaire brought tears to my eyes. The dedication and determination

shown by Susan and her husband were extra-
ordinary. Their success made me feel so glad that I
had written the Flat Stomach Plan.

## Pre-menstrual Tension

Sue Hill from Lancashire lost a stone in the first four
weeks and five inches from her waistline. She wrote:

'Normally I suffer from very bad pre-menstrual symptoms – mood swings, very sore breasts and a swollen
abdomen. I noticed that these were very much
reduced, especially the soreness in my breasts.'

Sue went on to say:

'Energy – I'm buzzing with it! I feel so much better
both mentally and physically.'

Margaret Howard from Derbyshire bought a copy of
the original Flat Stomach Plan book and whilst she
didn't need to lose very much weight – she was only
5ft 1in and weighed in at 8st 5lb before starting the
diet – she felt the healthy eating and exercises would
benefit her. Much to her surprise, whilst she only
lost three pounds during the first four weeks, she lost
three and a half inches from her waist and two and
three quarter inches from her abdomen. Margaret
wrote:

'Thank you for a great diet and exercise plan. I was
really surprised at the inches I have lost. I have actually enjoyed doing the exercises – even the children

have joined in with them. I have also been jogging, which is something I have never done in my life before. The best part of this plan is that it seems to have cured my pre-menstrual problems. For the last six years I have suffered from breast tenderness, feeling bloated, mood swings – the last six months have been the worst. I was having PMT symptoms 10 to 14 days before each period. The worst symptom was the breast tenderness. I was feeling really low and depressed.

'I have been on the diet and exercise plan for five weeks. During this time I have had a period with no PMT symptoms. To me it is like a small miracle. I have suffered for six years when all I needed to do was change my diet. I have tried to do this before by cutting out chocolate and junk food but I found this very hard.

'I have enjoyed being on this plan and I intend to stay with it. I feel so much better, like a new person. My husband and children have noticed a difference, especially in my mood. My husband has been marvellous. He has helped me and encouraged me and he loves my new figure. He also has given me £10 for every inch I have lost which amounts to £125 so far. Thank you once again for a new me.'

# Index of Recipes

# INDEX

## Activity Record Sheet

Keep a record of your daily activity and make a note of how you felt after the activity.

| DATE | ACTIVITY/EXERCISE | DURATION | COMMENTS |
|------|-------------------|----------|----------|
|      |                   |          |          |
|      |                   |          |          |
|      |                   |          |          |
|      |                   |          |          |
|      |                   |          |          |
|      |                   |          |          |

**Activity Record Sheet**

## Measurement Record Chart

| DATE | WEIGHT | BUST | WAIST | HIPS | WIDEST PART |
|------|--------|------|-------|------|-------------|
|      |        |      |       |      |             |
|      |        |      |       |      |             |
|      |        |      |       |      |             |
|      |        |      |       |      |             |
|      |        |      |       |      |             |
|      |        |      |       |      |             |
|      |        |      |       |      |             |
|      |        |      |       |      |             |
|      |        |      |       |      |             |
|      |        |      |       |      |             |
|      |        |      |       |      |             |
|      |        |      |       |      |             |
|      |        |      |       |      |             |
|      |        |      |       |      |             |
|      |        |      |       |      |             |
|      |        |      |       |      |             |
|      |        |      |       |      |             |
|      |        |      |       |      |             |
|      |        |      |       |      |             |
|      |        |      |       |      |             |

# MEASUREMENT RECORD CHART

| TOP OF THIGHS | | ABOVE KNEES | | UPPER ARMS | | COMMENTS |
|---|---|---|---|---|---|---|
| L | R | L | R | L | R | |
| | | | | | | |
| | | | | | | |
| | | | | | | |
| | | | | | | |
| | | | | | | |
| | | | | | | |
| | | | | | | |
| | | | | | | |
| | | | | | | |
| | | | | | | |
| | | | | | | |
| | | | | | | |
| | | | | | | |
| | | | | | | |
| | | | | | | |
| | | | | | | |
| | | | | | | |
| | | | | | | |

## Weight-loss Graph

Make up your own graph for each stone you lose,
following the example below.

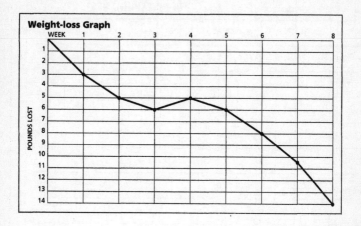

# WEIGHT-LOSS GRAPH

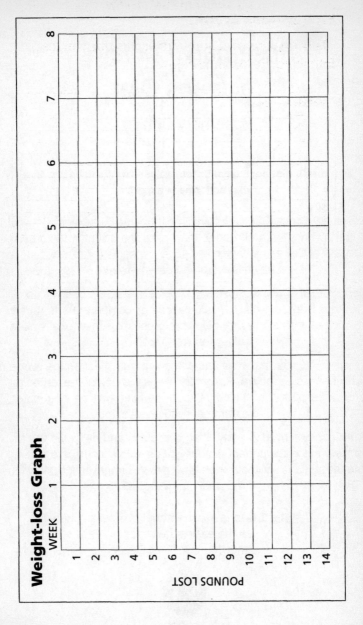

**Weight-loss Graph**

WEEK

POUNDS LOST

1 2 3 4 5 6 7 8

1
2
3
4
5
6
7
8
9
10
11
12
13
14

# *Rosemary Conley's Gi Jeans Diet*

## Rosemary Conley

**The new Gi diet book from Britain's best-loved and bestselling diet and fitness expert.**

Rosemary Conley CBE is Britain's most trusted diet expert. So who better to bring us a diet book that takes the scientifically proven success of Glycaemic Indexing (Gi) but presents it in a way that is straightforward and easy to follow.

Unlike other Gi books, *Rosemary Conley's Gi Jeans Diet* will do all the hard work for you. No calculations or complex charts, but a simple, easy to follow diet plan that promises sensational weight loss results – fast!

To maximise your progress and achieve a truly great shape everyone needs to get active. Rosemary brings you her best-ever toning excercises plus the choice of a fat-burning walking or running programme – you choose.

With a choice of tried and tested diet plans and delicious low fat recipes, this is the perfect diet for getting in to shape – and getting into those jeans – without even having to go hungry. It is healthy for the whole family too!

'I lost 2 stone 1 lb in 8 weeks without ever feeling hungry. It's the easiest diet ever'
Rodney Munns – Trial Dieter

arrow books

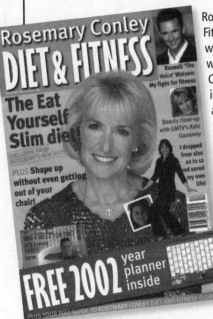

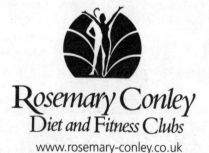

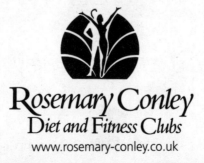

**Order further Rosemary Conley titles
from your local bookshop, or have them delivered
direct to your door by Bookpost**

---

| | | |
|---|---|---|
| ☐ **Gi Jeans Diet** | 0 09 949257 1 | £6.99 |
| ☐ **New Body Plan** | 0 09 944164 0 | £6.99 |
| ☐ **Complete Hip and Thigh Diet** | | |
| | 0 09 944162 4 | £6.99 |
| ☐ **New Inch Loss Plan** | 0 09 927102 8 | £12.99 |
| ☐ **Eat Yourself Slim** (Hardback) | 0 71 261553 9 | £12.99 |
| ☐ **Low Fat Cookbook** (Hardback) | 0 71 268462 X | £14.99 |

---

### Free post and packing

Overseas customers allow £2 per paperback

Phone: 01624 677237

Post: Random House Books
c/o Bookpost, PO Box 29, Douglas, Isle of Man IM99 1BQ

Fax: 01624 670923

email: bookshop@enterprise.net

Cheques (payable to Bookpost) and credit cards accepted

Prices and availability subject to change without notice.
Allow 28 days for delivery.
When placing your order, please state if you do not wish to receive any
additional information.

www.randomhouse.co.uk/arrowbooks

arrow books